Aktuelle Forschung Medizintechnik

Editor-in-Chief:
Th. M. Buzug, Lübeck, Deutschland

T0238441

Unter den Zukunftstechnologien mit hohem Innovationspotenzial ist die Medizintechnik in Wissenschaft und Wirtschaft hervorragend aufgestellt, erzielt überdurchschnittliche Wachstumsraten und gilt als krisensichere Branche. Wesentliche Trends der Medizintechnik sind die Computerisierung, Miniaturisierung und Molekularisierung. Die Computerisierung stellt beispielsweise die Grundlage für die medizinische Bildgebung, Bildverarbeitung und bildgeführte Chirurgie dar. Die Miniaturisierung spielt bei intelligenten Implantaten, der minimalinvasiven Chirurgie, aber auch bei der Entwicklung von neuen nanostrukturierten Materialien eine wichtige Rolle in der Medizin. Die Molekularisierung ist unter anderem in der regenerativen Medizin, aber auch im Rahmen der sogenannten molekularen Bildgebung ein entscheidender Aspekt. Disziplinen übergreifend sind daher Querschnittstechnologien wie die Nano- und Mikrosystemtechnik, optische Technologien und Softwaresysteme von großem Interesse.

Diese Schriftenreihe für herausragende Dissertationen und Habilitationsschriften aus dem Themengebiet Medizintechnik spannt den Bogen vom Klinikingenieurwesen und der Medizinischen Informatik bis hin zur Medizinischen Physik, Biomedizintechnik und Medizinischen Ingenieurwissenschaft.

Bernhard Gleich

Principles and Applications of Magnetic Particle Imaging

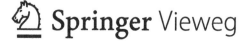
Springer Vieweg

Bernhard Gleich
University of Lübeck, Germany

Dissertation University of Lübeck, 2013

ISBN 978-3-658-01960-0   ISBN 978-3-658-01961-7 (eBook)
DOI 10.1007/978-3-658-01961-7

The Deutsche Nationalbibliothek lists this publication in the Deutsche Nationalbibliografie;
detailed bibliographic data are available in the Internet at http://dnb.d-nb.de.

Library of Congress Control Number: 2013945555

Springer Vieweg
© Springer Fachmedien Wiesbaden 2014

Printed on acid-free paper

Springer Vieweg is a brand of Springer DE.
Springer DE is part of Springer Science+Business Media.
www.springer-vieweg.de

Preface by the Series Editor

The book *Principles and Applications of Magnetic Particle Imaging* by Dr. Bernhard Gleich is the sixth volume of the new Springer-Vieweg series of excellent theses in medical engineering. The thesis of Dr. Gleich has been selected by an editorial board of highly recognized scientists working in that field.

The Springer-Vieweg series aims to establish a forum for Monographs and Proceedings on Medical Engineering. The series publishes works that give insights into the novel developments in that field.

Prospective authors may contact the Series Editor about future publications within the series at:

Prof. Dr. Thorsten M. Buzug
Series Editor Medical Engineering

Institute of Medical Engineering
University of Lübeck
Ratzeburger Allee 160
23562 Lübeck
Web: www.imt.uni-luebeck.de
Email: buzug@imt.uni-luebeck.de

Foreword

Bernhard Gleich and Jürgen Weizenecker published their revolutionary idea for Magnetic Particle Imaging (MPI), a novel medical imaging modality based on the direct interaction of iron-oxide nanoparticles with oscillating magnetic fields, in the Journal Nature in 2005. This was the starting point for a number of research groups around the world to implement the principle idea and to push forward the development of new designs concepts.

However, at that time Bernhard Gleich already made a head start since his first patent on MPI had been filed in 2001 — and he has used the first years of the century well for setting up the world-wide first 3D dynamical MPI small animal scanner. The 2005 Nature paper just summarized the work of the first years and showed a proof-of-concept. In the second half of this first decade, Bernhard Gleich and his co-workers published a number of key papers on MPI.

The scientific community in medical imaging reacted enthusiastic, because in the last three decades the matured imaging modalities, especially computed tomography (CT) and magnetic resonance imaging (MRI), have undergone some gradual technical improvements only. In contrast, magnetic particle imaging is based on a new physical principle and scanners must be build — up from the scratch. However, establishing a new modality is hard work and Bernhard Gleich accepted this challenge. This book summarizes the results of a number of original papers and countless innovations Bernhard Gleich has achieved in the young discipline of magnetic particle imaging — a discipline he has founded himself.

Prof. Dr. Thorsten M. Buzug
Institute of Medical Engineering
University of Lübeck

Contents

1 Introduction

This thesis aims at introducing Magnetic Particle Imaging (MPI), including all aspects that are necessary for a complete understanding. MPI is a new method for imaging the concentration of magnetic material. It was invented during the years 2000 and 2001.

The starting point for the deveopement of MPI was the fact that in MRI, only the magnetization determines the *possible* signal to noise ratio and not the frequency of recording. As MRI is very close to the physical optimum in recording, the only way to increase SNR or speed is to develope a method that utilizes a higher magnetization in the patient than the nuclear magnetization in MRI. It was evident that only ferromagnets could produce a much stronger magnetization than the proton magnetization in MRI. A method that is based on the detection of ferromagnetic material could become both fast and sensitive even at a high resolution. The next question was how to utilize the magnetization for imaging. The first, natural idea was to use ferromagnetic resonance and an MRI like encoding scheme. But it turned out that the technological challanges, especially in terms of particle properties, were discouragingly large. The next idea to analyze was to use Barkhausen jumps and a set of receiving coils to localize large magnetic particles e.g., in gastro-intestinal imaging. As a single jump occures at a specific location, it is possible to reconstruct the location of the event. This would work as long as the number of jumps is low. Imaging in a large object, like a human, would not work, as the jumps would start to overlap and the reconstruction of the event would fail. The next improvement step was to "switch off" a large fraction of the examined object by applying additional static fields. Field geometries with a field free point and a field free line are most efficient for this. These geometries allowed to omit the Barkhausen jumps and simply use the non-linearity of the magnetic material. Together with the idea of looking at the harmonics of a pure sine modulation or drive field, the basics of MPI were developed. The omission of the Barkhausen jumps allowed the use of iron oxide nano-particles as contrast agent (or tracer material). Injectable iron oxide nano-particles are available for MRI applications making medical applications for MPI much more likely. Therefore it was justified to file a patent application [Gle01] (published 2003) and to start a project to build a first demonstration model. In 2004, the scanner was in a state to produce images with reasonable quality and experimental results were published in 2005 [GW05].

Starting form the '2005 scanner', imaging sensitivity and speed continuously improved, patient access was enlarged, and it became possible to acquire images from living animals.

The following paragraphs give an outline of this thesis.

To set MPI into perspective and a context with established imaging methods, Chapter 2 introduces a classification scheme for medical imaging methods. This classification scheme is applied to some established and some novel medical imaging techniques and a set of properties is extracted that characterize successful imaging methods.

Chapter 3 describes the basic idea of MPI, including some technological aspects which are considered important for an actual implementation, and delivers a brief rollout of the image reconstruction.

As MPI won't deliver any image information without the use of a suitable magnetic material, Chapter 4 introduces the properties of magnetic particles, in particular two important concepts of the physics of magnetism, namely the demagnetizing field and magnetic domains, and dicusses their implications for MPI. Furthermore, the Langevin theory is introduced, together with its limitations, as a first, basic description of magnetic particle behaviour.

The introduction of the "focus field" in Chapter 5 completes the presentation of MPI. While the focus field is not essential for operating MPI, it is one possible solution to realizing an extended field of view and still maintain physiological compatibility.

After the introduction of MPI, Chapter 6 will focus on the analysis of imaging properties, i.e., spatial resolution, sensitivity, and temporal resolution, and how MPI compares to established methods for medical imaging.

After briefly summarizing the results of experimental studies and simulations in Chapter 7, Chapters 8 and 9 will give more details of the potential medical and non-medical applications. In particular, Chapter 8 discusses applications which are possible with systems and particles as described in the preceeding chapters, while Chapter 9 discusses applications which are only possible if the instrumentation and particles are improved or modified beyond their current status. While the nature of such applications might be speculative, their description can open the door for new directions in research on medical diagnosis and therapy.

Finally, Chapter 10 concludes this thesis, presenting an overview of all techniques in the context of MPI.

2 Medical imaging methods

The purpose of this chapter is to introduce a classification scheme for medical imaging methods. This is then applied to some established and some novel medical imaging techniques and a set of properties is extracted that characterizes successful imaging methods.

A "medical imaging method" can be defined as a method to image parts of a human or animal, e.g., to acquire data about the tissue, the tissue composition or characteristics, the bones, or even about physiological characteristics using special substances, called tracers, which are injected into the body. The region of interest can be inside the body, i.e., it can be several centimeters below any accessible surface. The scope of this document is limited to such methods, i.e. methods that image only the surface like thermography or only a few mm deep like optical coherence tomography are not discussed.

Established methods for clinical use, which should be discussed for any such scheme of characterization of medical imaging methods, are:

- X-ray imaging

- Computed Tomography (CT)

- UltraSound Imaging (US)

- Magnetic Resonance Imaging (MRI)

- Scintigraphy (Anger camera)

- Single Photon Emission Computed Tomography (SPECT)

- Positron Emission Tomography (PET)

Besides these, other methods, which are less common in clinical use or that are in experimental status, will be considered:

- Electrical Impedance Tomography

- Diffuse Optical Tomography

- Thermoacoustic/Photoacoustic Imaging

- Electron Paramagnetic Resonance Imaging (EPR)

This thesis will not explain how these methods work in detail, but rather focus on some common features involved in the characterization scheme. These aspects are signal penetration, tissue interaction, and signal confinement.

2.1 Signal penetration

To form an image of an area within a body, it is necessary for the signal to penetrate the tissue. Likewise, it is necessary to acquire the signal that is emitted by the tissue, i.e., information about the tissue. Consequently, it is necessary for any imaging method to use information carriers that penetrate human tissue for at least some centimeters, and preferably more. Table 2.1 lists signals and information carriers that have the ability to penetrate tissue sufficiently. As the inital signal entering the body (send signal) and the signal that carries the information about the tissue (emitted signal) do not need to be of the same type, it is possible to construct candidates for methods of medical imaging by combining one signal type as the send signal with another signal type as the receive signal. This way, one can theoretically construct 21 different medical imaging methods (some are left out, since methods in which *no* signal is emitted from the body do not make a reasonable imaging method—others are not possible for reasons given by the laws of nature).

Low frequency electromagnetic fields (**LF**) are well known from MRI. **X-rays** are the basis for X-ray imaging and computed tomography (CT), and accoustic waves **elast** are commonly used in ultrasound. Using light **OPT** or atomic particles **ptcl** is currently not common for medical imaging, but the underlying concepts are straightforward. They can be used in the same way as low frequency electromagnetic fields or X-rays.

The information carrier "fluidic matter" (**fluid**) needs some explanation. While the use of fluidic matter as a send signal initially seems

LF: Low frequency electromagnetic fields (0 Hz to about 1 GHz)

OPT: Optical / near infrared and red light (1.2 μm to 750 nm)

X-ray: X-rays, γ-rays (energies above $\approx$10 keV)

elast: Acoustic waves (0 Hz to $\approx$10 MHz)

ptcl: Particles at high energies (e.g., electrons, protons, neutrons and neutrinos)

fluid: Fluidic matter (e.g., something that can be injected using a syringe, e.g a nuclear tracer)

none: Special case: no signal enters the tissue, but the tissue itself emits signal

Table 2.1: Information carriers used in medical imaging

cryptic, it is actually quite common. One example would be the methods used in nuclear medicine (SPECT, PET), where a radioactive tracer is injected and is "fluidic matter". Another example, which is beyond what could be understand as a "fluid", would be a macroscopic device—to be more specific, it would be possible to acquire an image of a vessel tree by localizing the positions of an RF emitting marker on a catheter. The use of "fluidic matter" as an emitted signal to acquire information about the tissue is theoretically possible, but it is unlikely that it is actually used. A beam of X-rays with a very high intensity, for example, would damage the tissue and a change in the blood composition can be expected. So, theoretically, scanning the patient with the beam bit by bit and drawing and analysing many blood samples, could be used to make an image that would display information about certain tissue characteristics.

The information carrier "Nothing" can only be used in the sense of bringing nothing into the body, as it would, for example, be possible to collect low frequency electrical noise data to map the temperature of deep lying tissue. However, using "Nothing" as an emitted signal would most certainly not result in an image.

It is also possible to use two or more of these information carriers in combination. An example would be the injection of a contrast agent (e.g., fluid used as a send signal) and imaging with X-ray or MRI (e.g., LF or X-ray used as send and emitted signals).

2.2 Tissue interaction

Another essential feature of an imaging method is the interaction of the information carriers with the tissue[1]. This interaction has to vary with different tissues to generate a tissue specific contrast. Neutrinos, for example, are excellent in penetrating tissue, but the interaction is so low that imaging does not seem to be feasible.

Physics allows for a large number of interactions and it does not seem feasible to describe them all in detail. Nevertheless, the interactions can be classified into two categories:

- an intrinsic interaction with the tissue (without tracer or contrast agent) and

- an interaction with an injected contrast agent or tracer.

An example of the first category would be tissue specific absorption of X-rays, which yields an excellent visualization of bones. An example of the second category would be electron paramagnetic resonance imaging (EPR). The intrinsic concentration of free radicals is very low and an injected tracer generates essentially all the interaction.

For useful medial imaging, the contrast mechanism must be tissue specific. Again, two categories can be observed:

- the tissue specificity is intrinsic (i.e., no further help by tracers or contrast agents is needed)

- the tissue specificity has to be mediated by an injected contrast agent or tracer.

Staying within the example for the first category above, one can observe that bones have a much higher X-ray absorption than the surrounding soft tissue: therefore the excellent visualization of bones. On the other hand, and this constitutes an example for tissue specificity mediated by a tracer or contrast agent, X-ray absorption in blood is very similar to absorption in the vessel walls. Consequently, an X-ray

---

[1]Tissue in this context also refers to bones and anything else which is present within the body.

absorbing contrast agent is needed to generate a contrast that exposes the vessel lumen.

Taking it all together, the above categories can be combined to form four types of tissue interaction, as listed in Table 2.2.

1 Intrinsic interaction & intrinsic contrast. (e.g., ultrasound, MRI, X-ray, CT)

2 Intrinsic interaction & contrast agent modulates intrinsic interaction (e.g., contrast enhanced MRI)

3 Contrast agent mediated interaction & no tissue contrast agent interaction (e.g., contrast enhanced CT, angiography, hyperpolarized MRI)

4 Contrast agent mediated interaction & agent tissue interaction (e.g., O_2 sensing in EPR, hyperpolarized MRI [2])

Table 2.2: Four types of tissue interaction

Type 1 has the advantage of not needing any contrast agent, which simplifies the examination and workflow. Type 3 essentially images the pure concentration and distribution of a contrast agent, which has the potential to ease image interpretation. Types 2 and 4 have the capability to map tissue parameters.

2.3 Signal confinement/resolution

The third aspect used in characterizing imaging modalities is to look at how they confine the tissue interaction to a small volume. If the interaction is not confined, sufficient spatial resolution and image formation is not possible. There are several ways to confine the interaction[3], the three most important are listed in Table 2.3.

In **i**, at least one of the information carriers has be focused on a small region with a size on the order of the desired resolution. This is possible

---

[2]Hyperpolarized MRI is an example that is listed in 3 and 4, as it can use different nuclei and different chemical compounds with different imaging sequences.

[3]To form an image, the interaction does not need to be confined directly to the "voxel" of the image. It is also possible to confine the interaction to other geometries and compute the voxels from these resulting signals.

    i   geometrical and wave optics (e.g., X-ray, CT, ultrasound)

   ii near field methods (e.g., diffuse optical tomography, electrical impedance tomography)

  iii field-confined interaction (e.g., MRI)

Table 2.3: Methods to confine tissue interaction to small volumes

for X-rays, elastic waves of high enough frequency (e.g., >100 kHz for 1 cm resolution) and some particle rays.

In **ii**, the information carrier cannot be confined. Optical photons, for example, are heavily scattered in most tissues, so that signal propagation is a very diffusive process. Low frequency electromagnetic fields cannot be localized in deep lying tissue by using devices at the surface of the tissue. Still, theoretically, an image with arbitrary resolution can be reconstructed from data obtained at the surface. This can be easily understood in one dimension (cf. Fig. 6.1): The signal from one voxel is convolved with a smooth function. A convolution has an inverse function, as long as the Fourier coefficients do not drop to zero, which is the case for Gauss-like functions, even when very broad. Thus, a high-resolution image can be reconstructed when data are sampled on a fine grid at the surface of the patient. The problem is that the spatial Fourier components of the sampled data containing the high-resolution information rapidly drop to the noise floor. So in practice, resolution hardly reaches 1 cm. [4]

In **iii**, the problems of case **ii** are overcome by confining the interaction using a physical effect that is modulated by a field. This can also be understood as using an interaction with a non-linear response, i.e., doubling all fields in strength does not result in doubling the signal obtained. Exploiting this kind of interaction for spatial confinement was called "zeugmatography" by Lauterbur [Lau73]. The most prominent example is MRI and related techniques. Here, the resonance for a given frequency occurs only for a definite magnetic field. By applying a gradient field, the interaction is confined to a (curved) plane. Another example is the generation of harmonics in ultrasound imaging. As with

---

[4]Sometimes it is said that this is an *ill posed problem*. This is true, but misleading as e.g., the CT reconstruction is ill posed in the mathematical sense. Still CT images exhibit high resolution.

two-photon techniques in optical microscopy, the non-linear effect of the generation of harmonics strongly increases with the field strength, and therefore confines the interaction to a smaller spot in the focus.

2.4 Overview of existing imaging methods

This section categorizes established imaging methods by their use of information carriers (what type of signals they use), as well as their approach to tissue interaction (how do they generate a contrast) and signal confinement (how do they achieve spatial resolution). Table 2.4 presents the results of the categorization together with the "maturity" of the imaging method (is it already used for routine clinical imaging or is it still in a pre-clinical or even experimental state), which is displayed as a colour code.

One important observation is that there are many methods proposed or used for tomographic imaging in a medical context, but only a few have made it to routine clinical use. Another observation is that methods that utilize ionized, fast particles are rarely used for medical imaging: their use is limited to one method associated with heavy-ion therapy for oncology. The reason for the lack of particle based imaging modalities is probably the potential damage to tissue. Physical effects that involve sufficiently high energy to produce tissue-penetrating particles are also destructive to the tissue. Consequently, using them for general diagnostics is strongly discouraged.

One further observation is that no optical method has reached routine clinical use, although optical methods have good intrinsic tissue contrast and a variety of useful contrast agents exist for use in small animal imaging. Additionally, photoacoustic tomography is an optical method with reasonable resolution. The main problem with optical methods is the low tissue penetration of red and infrared light, which limits their use. The light intensity is reduced to roughly 10% for every cm of tissue. Thus, imaging deeper than 5 cm becomes challenging and at a depth of 10 cm, virtually no photon can penetrate the tissue and return to the surface. Consequently, applications in adult humans are limited mainly to the limbs and the female breast. In the light of such limited potential applications, the economic risks in developing an optical imaging method for clinical use may seem too high.

Furthermore, it is also interesting to notice that no method without

	LF	OPT	X-ray	elast
LF	**MRI (iii,1,2)**^{4} *EIT (ii,1)*^{3} MIT (ii,1)^1 H-MRI (iii,3,4)^2 O-MRI (iii,4)^2			*TAT (i,1)*^{3} MAT (i,1)^1 MAT-MI (i,1)^1
OPT		*DOT (ii,1,3,4)*^{3} UMOT (i,1,3,4)^2		PAT (i,1,3,4)^2
X-ray			**X-ray (i,1,3)**^{4} **CT (i,1,3)**^{4} **DSA (i,3)**^{4} CSCT (i,1)^2	XAT (i,1,3)^1
elast	MAET (i,1)^1	SLI (i,1,3,4)^1		**US (i,1,3)**^{4} **HI (i,1,3)**^{4}
ptcl			**ITM (i,1)**^{4}	
fluid			**SZG (i,3)**^{4} **SPECT (i,3)**^{4} **PET (i,3)**^{4}	
none	*MTI (ii,1)*^{3}	*BLI (ii,1)*^{3}		PTT (i,1)^1

^{4}: **Clinically used**
^{3}: *Images in human shown*
^{2}: In vivo images shown
^{1}: In vitro experiments/method proposed

Table 2.4: A selection of established imaging modalities classified by their use of information carriers, their approach to tissue interaction, given arabic numbers as listed in Table 2.2, and signal confinement, given in roman numbers as listed in Table 2.3. The superscripts and the font indicate the maturity of the method. The acronyms used for the imaging methods are listed in Tables 2.5 to 2.7.

a good (type **i** and **iii**) way of confining the tissue interaction to a small volume has reached routine clinical use. A deconvolution of diffusion equations or static Maxwell equations yields resolutions no better than 2 cm in deep tissue. Given such a resolution, only large lesions can be detected, which limits the practical clinical use.

All diagnostic imaging methods used in a clinical context rely on or can be improved by the use of a contrast agent. The use of an injected fluid results in additional contrast with potentially high clinical relevance.

From Table 2.4 it can be observed that elastic waves have a high

MRI: Magnetic Resonance Imaging A strong magnetic field is applied together with a small gradient. A radio-frequency pulse is applied which matches the resonance condition of, e.g., one slice. The "echo" of the resonance is measured while being modulated by the change of gradients. [Lau73]

EIT: Electrical Impedance Tomography The AC electrical impedance between electrodes is measured. [TOK08]

MIT: Magnetic Induction Tomography The magnetic field of eddy currents in tissue is measured. [MHOS04]

DOT: Diffuse Optical Tomography The propagation of light between a collection of points on the tissues surface is measured. [CCL+05]

X-ray: X-ray Projection Imaging The X-ray photons transmitted through the tissue from a point source are displayed. [Rön96]

CT: X-ray Computed Tomography A slice or volume is irradiated with X-rays from many angles and a 2D or 3D image is computed from the transmitted rays. [Hou73]

US: UltraSound Imaging Tissue is irradiated with a focused ultrasound beam and the reflected and scattered ultrasound is measured. [Dus42]

SPECT: Single Photon Emission Computed Tomography A gamma-ray emitter (tracer) is brought into the patient and the emitted photons are collimated and measured. As in CT, the collimated photons are collected from many angles and a 3D image is reconstructed. [KE63]

PET: Positron Emission Tomography A positron emitter (tracer) is brought into the patient. The two annihilation photons are detected in coincidence and the direction of emission is deduced. From the ensemble of these emission directions, a 3D image is computed. [TPPHM75] [CHB73]

PAT: PhotoAcoustic Tomography Red or near infrared light heats the tissue. The tissue expands and thereby emits an acoustic wave. [ZLC+08]

TAT: ThermoAccoustic Tomography A radio wave heats the tissue. The tissue expands and thereby emits an acoustic wave. [KMR+00]

Table 2.5: Abbreviations as used in Table 2.4, together with a a short explanation and references.

potential of interacting with other information carriers. They can be produced by any information carrier by a thermoacoustic effect (even if no known imaging modalities exist).

Although thermoacoustic tomography breast images have been demonstrated with a quality comparable to or even exceeding those

BLI: BioLuminescence Imaging The weak chemo- bio-luminescence of tissue metabolism is measured. [EIJKT90]

SZG: SZintiGraphy The X-ray (gamma-ray) photons from an injected tracer are collimated and detected. [Ang58]

H-MRI: Hyperpolarized MRI Hyperpolarized MRI is like MRI, but the measured magnetization is introduced to the tissue by the injection/inhalation of externally hyperpolarized material. [GKD^{+}08]

O-MRI: Overhauser Overhauser enhanced magnetic resonance works like MRI, but the magnetization of the nuclei is increased by the use of a double-resonance with unpaired electrons. [HMM^{+}08]

DSA: Digital Subtraction Angiography Contrast enhanced X-ray projection imaging, where the image without contrast agent is subtracted. [CSS^{+}80] [OCF^{+}80]

MAT: MagnetoAcoustic Tomography A current is applied to the tissue. In an additional static magnetic field, the current leads to Lorentz forces, which give rise to ultrasound emissions. The ultrasound is detected. [RBW94]

MAT-MI: MagnetoAcoustic Tomography with Magnetic Induction Works like MAT, but the current is not fed to the tissue by electrodes, but by a time-varying magnetic field [YB05].

PTT: Passive Thermoacoustic Tomography The acoustic noise emitted by the tissue is recorded. [PAB00]

ITM: Heavy Ion Therapy Monitoring The distribution of positron emitters produced by heavy ion therapy is imaged using positron emission tomography [PBH08]

Table 2.6: Abbreviations as used in Table 2.4 (continued)

of classical ultrasound imaging, a clinical use does not seem apparent. Possible reasons may be the intrinsic limitations of ultrasound: It does not penetrate the lung and has problems near bones and the (gas filled) intestine. In consequence, a large part of the body is not accessible. An additional problem is that the complex mechanical properties of the tissue (diffraction, scattering, attenuation) significantly limit the practical resolution. Improvements can be expected if the tissue to be imaged is accessible from many angles. Thus practically, thermoacoustic methods are also limited to the limbs and the female breast, which may limit the potential market.

SLI: SoloLuminiscence Imaging High intensity focused ultrasound produces collapsing bubbles leading to thermal light emission. [HXT+02]

UMOT: Ultrasound Modulated Optical Tomography The propagation of light in tissue is measured, while an ultrasound wave modulates the local optical properties. [YW00]

MAET: Magneto-Acousto-Electrical Tomography A focused ultrasound in the tissue produces a voltage dipole in a static magnetic field. The voltage at the surface of the tissue is measured. [HHX08]

XAT: X-ray Acoustic Tomography A pencil-beam X-ray flash heats the tissue. The tissue expands thermally and emits sound. [Bow82]

MTI: Microwave Thermometry Imaging The thermal microwave emissions of the tissue are measured. [LBM98]

HI: Harmonic Imaging The reflected higher harmonics of a ultrasound pulse are measured. [HHK98]

CSCT: Coherent Scatter Computed Tomography Scattered X-ray photons are measured in a geometry similar to X-ray computed tomography. [HKN87]

Table 2.7: Abbreviations as used in Table 2.4 (end)

2.5 Conclusions for successful new imaging modalities

It is now possible to discuss the requirements for building a successful imaging method, based on the observations included in the above sections of this chapter.

- The imaging method needs a good resolution, resulting from a type **i** or type **iii** encoding mechanism.

Any new method without a good spatial resolution will find a strong competitor in the well established nuclear methods. They realize excellent tissue contrast due to the wide range of available radiopharmaceuticals. In addition, MRI is also a strong competitor. For an application that is feasible with a low resolution, MRI would be fast and cheap. A very low resolution MRI image with 1 cm voxel size is acquired within seconds. So, there is not much room for a new low resolution imaging method.

- The imaging method must be able to image at least 10 cm, probably 20 cm deep inside the tissue.

By violating this requirement, the number of relevant applications decreases drastically. However, an imaging method without this ability might still be useful for special applications. Consequently, low frequency electromagnetic waves, X-rays and elastic waves seem to be the most promising information carriers.

- A new imaging method should have the ability to employ a contrast agent.

The use of contrast agents offers a broad range of applications that are otherwise difficult or impossible to address, e.g., dynamical aspects of the inflow and outflow of blood.

- A new imaging method should address a broad range of diseases.

All the existing successful imaging methods have a broad range of possible applications, including cardiology, oncology and neurology.
Besides these requirements, there are other properties of medical imaging methods that can be considered a "wish list".

* Avoid ionizing radiation

Ionizing radiation, e.g., X-rays, is perceived to be a hazard for the patient. It also imposes the need for safety equipment and procedures, thus complicating workflow and patient handling.

* Contrast without the use of a contrast agent

Although the ability to use an imaging method together with a contrast agent is believed to be one mandatory requirement (see above), it would still be benefical that an intrinsic contrast can be acquired without the use of a contrast agent. In the end, this would simplify workflow, patient handling and scan planning.

* If a contrast agent is to be used, then one with low toxicity

The injection of a contrast agent is always a risk to the patient, so it is desirable to use one that has low side effects at approved clinical dosages. This can also simplify the workflow, because in the case of a failed image acquisition, the contrast agent can be re-injected.

* High imaging speed

* Low cost

High speed and low cost are somewhat linked. If the speed of an imaging method is high, many patients can be scanned per day, thus distributing the cost of the scanner. On the other hand, high scanning speed allows for dynamic imaging which is of paramount importance for cardiovascular applications.

In the next chapters, Magnetic Particle Imaging (MPI) will be explained in detail; given the classification scheme of medical imaging methods and the requirements derived in this chapter, they will, of course, be applied to MPI and it will be checked whether MPI has the potential to become a successful new medical image modality.

3 Basic idea of Magnetic Particle Imaging

3.1 Signal generation and recording

The basic idea of magnetic particle imaging is described in brief in [GW05]. Here a more elaborate description shall be given.

To invent magnetic particle imaging (MPI), two ideas had to be combined. The first one is a method to detect a magnetic material using its non-linear magnetization curve. The second idea is to localize the detection using a magnetic field having a field free point. First I will concentrate on the detection of the magnetic material.

3.1.1 Signal generation

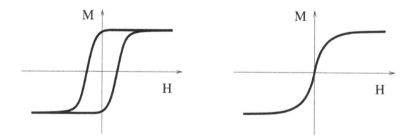

Figure 3.1: Magnetization curves with hysteresis (left) and without hysteresis (right).

A ferromagnetic material[1] can have a variety of magnetization curves usually displaying a hysteresis as sketched in the left graph of Fig. 3.1.

---

[1]this term will also be used for ferrimagnetic materials

For the explaination of MPI it is sufficient to neglect the hysteresis. Therefore, a magnetization curve as displayed in the right graph is assumed. At a low magnetic field strength, the magnetization increases linearly with the applied field strength. At higher fields, the increase in magnetization gets lower and the magnetization reaches a saturation level.

A magnetized material produces a magnetic field that can be detected using some kind of magnetometer. From magnetic resonance imaging it is known that a magnetization can be measured with equal sensitivity regardless of the frequency with which the magnetization changes [LL99]. When the magnetization oscillates faster, the induced voltage in a recording coil increases, so the signal strength rises with the frequency. On the other hand, the thermal current fluctuations due to the conductivity of the patient are frequency independent. For higher frequencies, these frequency independent currents generate a higher noise voltage in the recording coil, as faster fluctuations induce more voltage. In total the signal to noise ratio stays (almost) constant, independent of the chosen frequency of oscillation. This fact is also the reason why the signal to noise ratio in MRI is "only" proportional to the main field strength, i.e., the magnetization.

So for a first estimate of the detection limit for ferromagnetic materials, the typical measurable dipole moments in MRI can be compared to the dipole moment of small amounts of iron oxide. $1\,mm^3$ water at $1.5\,T\mu_0^{-1}$ has a dipole moment of about $5\,pAm^2$ and can be rapidly detected. So it is safe to assume a detection limit in MRI of well below $1\,pAm^2$. $10\,pg$ of iron oxide (magnetite) also has a dipole moment of about $1\,pAm^2$. Therefore, the detection limit for ferromagnetic material should lie below $10\,pg$, which would fit in a cube of roughly $(1\,\mu m)^3$, considerably smaller than for the MRI case.

The challenge of measuring the magnetization of a ferromagnetic material is twofold: The first challenge is the frequency of the magnetization change. If it is too low, the noise induced by the thermal field fluctuations around the patient is no more the limiting factor. Instead, the intrinsic noise of the detector, e.g., coil resistance or amplifier noise, dominates the noise. Therefore it is necessary to change the magnetization fast enough. The second challenge is the presence of the field to magnetize the ferromagnetic material. To change the magnetization of the magnetic material, fields in the order of $10\,mT\mu_0^{-1}$ may be needed. On the other hand the fields generated by the $10\,pg$ iron oxide, discussed above, are only of the order of $0.1\,\mathrm{fT}\mu_0^{-1}$. The ratio between the applied field and the detected field is therefore up to 10^{14}. This ratio clearly exceeds the dynamic range of common magnetometers, so special techniques are needed to be able to measure the magnetization change of the magnetic material.

The solution used in MRI is not applicable for magnetic material detection. In MRI, a short pulse of radio frequency magnetic field is applied to produce an echo in the spin system. This means the sample has an oscillating magnetization, while no alternating magnetic field is applied to the sample. Therefore, the magnetization can be measured without background and the dynamic range is not the limiting factor.

For the detection of magnetic material a similar technique exists. It is the basis of the magnetic marker monitoring technique (MMM [WKCT97] [WCK+99]). It uses the fact that the magnetization of some magnetic particles has a remanence, i.e., the magnetization persists for some time, even if no magnetic field is applied any more. So particles with a hysteresis (Fig. 3.1, left) are needed. This makes it possible to measure the magnetization without the applied field, but has the drawback that the frequencies involved are low. It takes at least some milliseconds until thx e eddy currents have decayed. So only processes with frequencies below $1\,\mathrm{kHz}$ can be observed. This makes superconducting recording elements necessary. In addition, it is not compatible with the spatial encoding scheme in MPI.

Another way to avoid the background is to use a detector configuration that is insensitive to the external field. An example of this is the gradiometer coils in SQUID magnetometers [CB04]. A change in the external magnetic field does not induce a current in the coil, but a change in sample magnetization does. This technique is compatible with MPI, but has a high burden of adjusting the detector, so its use for medical imaging may be limited.

The technique used in MPI relies on the non-linearity of the magnetization curve. The magnetization does not follow the external field proportionally. So the signal from the sample can be distinguished from the external field. An efficient way to implement this in electronics is to use a perfect sine as excitation and to look at the higher harmonics of the detected signal as depicted in Fig. 3.2. A perfect sine H field wave is applied to the magnetic material. In principle, a perfect sinusoidal field is generated by a resonant LC circuit. The magnetization M of the material is no longer a sine wave, but the magnetic field generated

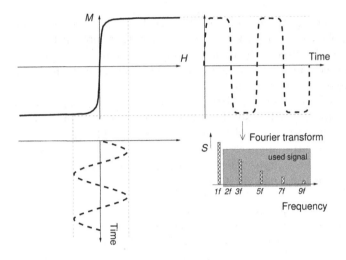

Figure 3.2: Generation of harmonics using a magnetic material.

by the magnetization is usually small and thus the total H field is still pretty close to a perfect sine. The superimposed sine is usually orders of magnitude higher than the field produced due to the magnetic material. Nevertheless, the harmonics in the magnetization signal can be detected in Fourier space. It is possible to suppress the fundamental frequency by LC tank circuits (notch filters).

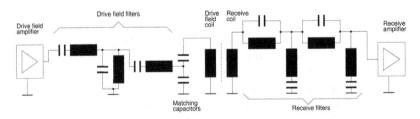

Figure 3.3: An example of a send and receive system for MPI. The signal is synthesized and fed to the drive field amplifier.

In Fig. 3.3, a circuit diagram of a send and receive filter implementation is sketched. The signal is synthesized and fed to the drive field amplifier. The harmonics of the amplifier are filtered by a band-pass filter. The number of stages depends on the purity of the signal at the drive field amplifier. The drive field coil is resonantly matched. The receive coil is coupled to the drive field coil, so the signal in the send-band has to be blocked in the receive chain. In addition, the impedance of the receive chain has to be high in the drive field band. Otherwise the receive could not be penetrated by the drive field. The number of stages in the receive band-stop filter depends on the linearity of the receive amplifier.

3.1.2 Signal confinement

After explaining how small quantities of magnetic material can be detected, it is now necessary to discuss how to confine the interaction to a small region. The simplest solution would be to apply the the magnetizing field only in a small volume. It turns out that this is impossible with low frequency electromagnetic fields as the static Maxwell equations allow no point with high field strength while, on a surface around the point, the field strength at any point is lower (no sources are allowed within the volume enclosed by the surface). So selective magnetization is not an option for imaging deep within the patient.

Instead, the Maxwell equations allow for a different "special point". Within a source-free region, it is possible to generate a point with zero field strength, while the field strength at all other points is non-zero (see Fig. 3.4). Electrical currents with opposite directions in two coils generate a magnetic field as sketched in the figure. The field lines do not reach the symmetric point of the assembly. Therefore the there is point of zero field strength. This point is called the "field free point" (FFP). The magnitude of the magnetic field increases in all directions from the field free point. In the vertical direction, the gradient of the magnitude is double that in the orthogonal directions. Coupling the signal generation to this field free point would allow good resolution in deep lying tissue.

To understand this coupling, it is beneficial to have a closer look at the generation of harmonics. As already seen in Fig. 3.2, if the average field is zero, it is possible to generate harmonics by applying a sinusoidal "modulation field". But, if a time-constant field is added on top of this modulation field (Fig. 3.5), the modulation field changes the magnetization only in the constant part of the magnetization curve.

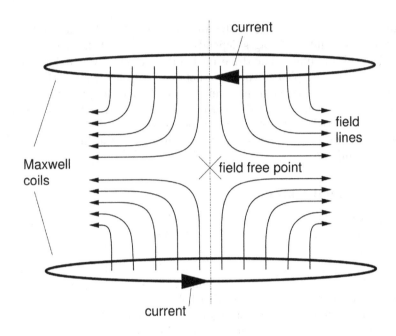

Figure 3.4: Maxwell coil assembly.

Therefore, no detectable signal is generated.

Now, the two ingredients can be combined to facilitate the spatial encoding. In the field with the FFP, called "selection field", the magnetic material is in a state of saturation. Therefore, the magnetization does not change and no higher harmonics are produced. Only near the FFP, the modulation field changes the magnetization significantly and only there are harmonics generated.

Forming an 3D image with this idea is straight-forward. The field free point is moved step by step over the object. At each position, a modulation field is applied and the amplitude of the harmonics is recorded. This amplitude is converted to a grey value for the corresponding voxel in the image. The movement of the FFP over the sample can be accomplished in different ways:

1. The sample is moved.

2. The scanner is moved.

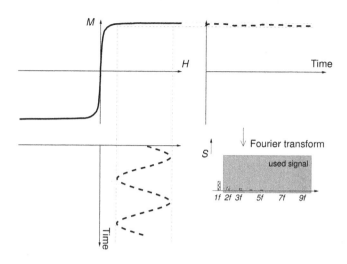

Figure 3.5: A time-constant field is added to the sine field wave.

3. Additional homogeneous fields move the FFP.

3.1.3 Drive field

The third option needs further explanation. If the FFP is moved to a specific position, the same field value originally found on this position has to be applied with the opposite direction in each component. The field shape near this new FFP is similar to the field shape at the original position. In fact, the Maxwell equations do not allow many different field shapes around a FFP. If the selection were a perfect homogeneous gradient field, the shape would stay exactly the same.

The option of being able to move the FFP by a homogeneous field has further implications. The modulation field is a more or less homogeneous field, so it will move the field free point. If the modulation field is weak, there will be only a small movement. But by increasing it, the movement will become larger and the argument of generation the signal only at the field free point breaks down.

In a later section it will be explained why a modulation field with a high amplitude is essential for efficient MPI imaging. As this high amplitude modulation field is so important, it was named the "drive

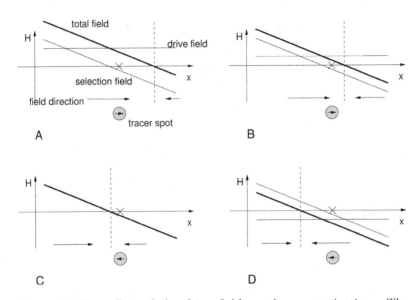

Figure 3.6: The effect of the drive field on the magnetization. The cross in the graphs indicates the position of the magnetic material and the dashed vertical line the position of the field free point. From A to D, the drive field value decreases. Therefore the position of the field free point moves over the spot with tracer material. Then, the field direction changes and the magnetization is reverted.

field". Signal generation using a drive field can be visualized as in Fig. 3.6. Assume the field free point moves with constant speed over a tiny spot with magnetic material. Before the FFP reaches the spot, the field direction at the spot position has one direction. After the FFP has moved past the spot, the field points in the opposite direction. So the magnetization changes direction when the FFP moves over the spot of magnetic material and, in turn, a voltage pulse is induced in the recording coil. This explanation assumes a magnetic material with a magnetization that instantaneously follows the external magnetic field. This in some sense "ideal" material has a step-like magnetization curve. Realistic magnetic material produces a less localized peak, resulting in a finite resolution.

In the introduction of the drive field above, the field free point is moved and pulses are generated and recorded. Still it is necessary to separate the pulses from the induced voltage due to the drive field. To separate the pulses from the drive field, it is still beneficial to use a perfect sine to move the FFP. The pulses have high Fourier components, thus they are readily separated by analog and digital filtering of the drive field frequency.

Due to the harmonic oscillation of the drive field, the field free point moves with different speeds over different locations. Therefore, the heights of the pulses differ depending on the location. When forming an image, these differences have to be corrected. This is one reason why a mathematical reconstruction process is needed in MPI.

3.2 Reconstruction

After having acquired the signal generated with the help of the drive field, an image has to be calculated, i.e., reconstructed. The simplest idea is to "track" the position of the FFP at any time and insert the magnitude of the induced voltage in a recording coil as a grey value in the corresponding voxel in the image. This procedure fails. It fails not only for real magnetic material, where, e.g., hysteresis would break the simple correlation between FFP position and signal generation position. It also fails for an ideal magnetic material with a magnetization direction instantaneously following the external magnetic field.

The reason for this failure can be seen in Fig. 3.7. Here a spot of ideal magnetic material is placed in the center. The FFP moves near and over the sample and the corresponding signal intensity is displayed. While the signal is well localized in the movement direction, the lateral extension is considerable. E.g., using z-magnetization and z-modulation (Fig. 3.7), the direct image of a spot would look like the upper-left image in the figure. Having two close by spots, the intensity of the blurring will add, as they will overlap. So, the appearance of the image will become more blurry. For continuous distributions of magnetic material, the blurring effect becomes even more prominent. This effect leads to strongly blurred images, if no reconstruction is applied.

The reason for the large extension in the vertical direction is the field geometry. It is best understood in the plane through the FFP where the field vector always points to the FFP (the plane with the lowest gradient strength). The magnetization of the ideal magnetic material has always

z-Modulation   x-Modulation

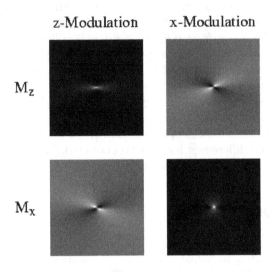

70nm Partikel, 1T/m Gradient

Figure 3.7: Signal amplitude generated near a spot of magnetic material. In the center, a simulated (Langevin theory) sample is
placed. In the z-modulation images, the FFP moves from
top to bottom over the image, in the x-modulation from left
to right, with constant speed. In the upper row, the derivative of the up-down magnetization is displayed; in the lower
row, the derivative of the horizontal magnetization.

saturation value, i.e., constant length and points to the FFP. If the FFP
moves directly over the magnetic material, the magnetization changes
instantaneously. This is the central high-intensity spot in Fig. 3.7. If
the FFP passes the magnetic material nearby, the change is still fast.
The main change in vertical magnetization takes place when the FFP
movement, seen from the magnetic material position, covers an angle of
about 90° symmetrically. As the direction of the magnetization vector
points to the FFP, it also rotates by 90°. So the magnetization in the
direction of FFP movement changes by $\sqrt{1/2}$. If the FFP passes the
magnetic material at a greater distance, it needs more time to cover the

angle. Thus the magnetization change is slower in the signal intensity (induced voltage) lower. The maximum intensity in horizontal direction drops only with $1/|x|$, x being the distance from the center. For most imaging applications, this intensity drop is too low to generate sharp images.

To generate an image without this blurring, a reconstruction algorithm has to be employed. The basic mathematics for an MPI reconstruction is relatively simple, as MPI is a good approximation to a linear imaging method. Linear means that if any (local) concentration in the sample is doubled, its effect on the generated signal is doubled. This condition is fulfilled in MPI as long as the fields generated by the magnetization are much smaller than the field needed to saturate the magnetic material.

In any linear imaging method, a reconstruction can be performed using the following recipe:

- move a small test sample to a position in space

- apply a "sequence" and measure the receive signal; store the test signal

- repeat the above steps until all voxels in the field of view have their associated stored signal

- insert the object with unknown "signal generator" distribution and apply the same sequence as in the steps before; store the object signal

- generate a weighted sum of the test signals and compare it to the object signal; vary the weighting coefficients to achieve the "best fit"

- the weight coefficients are the grey values of the corresponding image of the object.

In this context, a "sequence" is the time series of external fields applied to the objects. For MPI, this would be the path of the FFP. In a simple realization, he "best fit" can mean the smallest deviation between measured and fitted signal. Often it is necessary to add penalties for too high voxel to voxel variations in the weight coefficients. This is known as "regularization" [WTVF92].

The recipe for reconstruction can be formulated more mathematically: During a sequence, k values (e.g., voltages over time) are measured. Measuring the object, one measured value is called $U_n, n \in 1...k$. There are l positions at which the test sample is measured. Again, each measurement at one position produces k values. Then G_{nj} is an element of the so-called system function (in matrix representation) with $n \in 1...k$ and $j \in 1...l$. At the position j, the measured object has a concentration C_j. Therefore the expected signal component is:

$$U_n^{\text{exp}} = \sum_j G_{nj} C_j$$

This can also be written using vector notation:

$$\vec{U}^{\text{exp}} = \vec{G}\vec{C}$$

Where $\vec{G}$ is the matrix containing the values of the test measurement (system function). In the reconstruction step, $\vec{C}$ has to be varied to minimize $||\vec{U} - \vec{U}^{\text{exp}}||$, i.e.:

$$||\vec{U} - \vec{G}\vec{C}|| = \min$$

For the Euclidean norm, $\vec{C}$ can be computed as:

$$\vec{C} = \vec{G}^{-1}U$$

Simply computing the inverse of the system function and multiplying it by the measured vector usually fails as the measured data are usually noisy and due to other experimental shortcomings (drift, object motion, ...). In most cases some sort of regularization is needed. A regularization can be viewed as an *a priori* knowledge of the object. *A priori* knowledges may be a total concentration limit, or the exclusion of negative concentrations. The most frequently used *a priori* knowledge is a kind of smoothness of the concentration. More information on regularization can be found in [WTVF92].

The components of the vector $\vec{U}$ can consist of different measured quantities (voltages, currents, power over time) or derived quantities (Fourier transform, Chebyshev transform, ...). Using the measured quantities directly would be simple. But currently, the Fourier transformed voltages are mainly used. The reason is that the Fourier space allows for better preprocessing of the data. It is possible to reduce the number of values by discarding low and high frequency components. It is also possible to weight the different frequency values. This is useful, as additional harmonics are generated by the scanner and therefore have a high noise level.

4 Magnetic particle properties

In the previous section, it was assumed that some magnetic material exists which has a steep magnetization curve. Here, a brief introduction to the topic of the magnetism of small particles will be given and the properties of particles suitable for MPI will be described. Everything in this section can also be found in textbooks about magnetism such as [CC78] [Gob87] [Kit86]. But here only the most relevant aspects for MPI are summarized.

4.1 Demagnetization factor

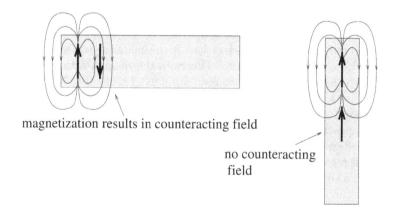

magnetization results in counteracting field

no counteracting
field

Figure 4.1: Origin of the demagnetization factor.

Looking into material databases it is easily possible to find soft magnetic material that saturates at a few $\mu T \mu_0^{-1}$. Having a gradient of $1\,T\mu_0^{-1}/m$ in the selection field, this would lead to resolutions on the order of a few μm. Unfortunately, this does not apply to compact

objects, such as particles. The reason for this is the so-called demagnetization factor. To explain this effect it is illustrative to assume a
perfectly soft magnetic material. This material has a saturation magnetization of $1\,\mathrm{T}\mu_0^{-1}$ and is shaped as a disk with infinite extensions
in the plane (Fig. 4.1, left). Assume for the moment that the mate-
rial consists of "spins" or "domains", i.e., small volumes that orient
themselves always completely in the direction of the field they "see".
Applying only a small external field perpendicular to the plane, e.g.,
$1\,\mu\mathrm{T}\mu_0^{-1}$, one could think that all these domains are oriented in the perpendicular direction. But now, we have to consider the magnetic field
of all the other "domains" at the position of one selected domain. In
a disk (left of the figure) an oriented magnetic dipole generates a field
in neighbouring areas that counters the magnetization direction of the
first dipole. From the figure it can be seen that this field is in the opposite direction to the first applied field. A calculation would reveal that
the field strength at the selected domain is $-1\,\mathrm{T}\mu_0^{-1}$. This means, the
domain has to flip immediately. This flipping has to happen also with
other domains statistically until almost an even distribution between
"up" and "down" orientation is reached. This generates a feedback
mechanism that weakens the magnetization in an external magnetic
field. The small $1\,\mu\mathrm{T}\mu_0^{-1}$-field leads only to a few net domains end-
ing oriented up. The magnetization of the material turns out to be
$1\,\mu\mathrm{T}\mu_0^{-1}$, i.e., the applied field. Therefore the magnetization curve is
not steep. Saturation is only reached at an external field of $1\,\mathrm{T}\mu_0^{-1}$, i.e.,
the saturation magnetization of the material. So harmonics are only
produced if the drive field has an amplitude higher than $1\,\mathrm{T}\mu_0^{-1}$ which
is an impractically large field.

The effect of demagnetization of a general shape is complicated, as
different regions reach saturation at different applied field strength. For
ellipses, a simple theory exists. Ellipses have a well defined "demagnetization factor" for each main axis. The magnetization at an external
field H of an ellipse of perfectly soft material and a demagnetization
factor N is:

$$M = \frac{H}{N}$$

In addition, the sum of the demagnetization factors of the three orthogonal directions is 1, i.e., $N_x + N_y + N_z = 1$. So, for a sphere
the demagnetization factor must be $1/3$. For an infinite long rod, the
demagnetization factor in the long direction is 0, and the orthogonal

Dimensional Ratio	Rod	Prolate Ellipsoid	Oblate Ellipsoid
0	1	1	1
1	0.27	0.3333	0.3333
2	0.14	0.1735	0.2364
5	0.040	0.0558	0.1248
10	0.0172	0.0203	0.0696
20	0.00617	0.00675	0.0369
50	0.00129	0.00144	0.01472
100	0.00036	0.000430	0.00776
200	0.000090	0.000125	0.00390
500	0.000014	0.0000236	0.001567
1000	0.0000026	0.0000066	0.000784
2000	0.0000009	0.0000019	0.000392

Table 4.1: The demagnetization factors of an oblate and prolate ellipse and the approximate demagnetization factor of a rod from [CC78].

demagnetization factors are 1/2. When magnetizing a rod in the long direction (Fig. 4.1, right), there are no net counteracting fields on neighbouring dipoles. Therefore the magnetization curve can be steep.

A small demagnetization factor leads to a strong magnetization and saturation at weak fields. For a small demagnetization factor, the shape must be elongated in at least one dimension and thin it at least one other. So needles and disks are well suited to produce a good resolution in MPI. For medical imaging, a saturation at a field of about $1\,\mathrm{mT}\mu_0^{-1}$ is needed. Typical magnetic material has a saturation value of $1\,\mathrm{T}\mu_0^{-1}$ and therefore a demagnetization factor of 10^{-3} is needed. From Table 4.1 it can be seen that needles with an aspect ratio of 1/100 are needed. Currently it is not clear if such needles can be manufactured in a way that they can be tolerated in a medical imaging application.

4.2 Single domain particles and the Langevin theory

It is not clear whether a contrast agent consisting of small needles or disks would be physiologically tolerable. But it is known that small iron oxide particles are tolerable when injected into humans. These are already available as contrast agents for MRI. But nearly spherical particles have a demagnetization factor of $1/3$ and are expected to saturate at a few hundred $mT\mu_0^{-1}$. The reason why these particles can serve as MPI contrast agents lies in the special magnetic properties of "single domain particles".

A ferromagnetic material consists of several magnetic domains in which the spins are oriented in parallel. Between different domains, domain walls exist. To form a domain wall, a material-dependent amount of energy per wall area is needed. On the other hand, energy is stored in the field around a domain. A part of the energy can be released by breaking the domain into two and orienting the magnetizations of the two domains anti-parallel. This energy gain is proportional to the third power of the domains' linear dimensions, while the wall energy is proportional to the square. Therefore a very small particle will not form domains, as there is not enough potential energy to form a single domain. These particles are called "single domain particles".

Such a single domain particle may be viewed as a tiny permanent magnet. If the magnetization can freely rotate, as when suspended in liquid, it will follow the external field as a compass needle does. So, a suspension of ferromagnetic single domain particles can saturate at low external magnetic fields.

There is a thermodynamic reason why saturation does not occur at an arbitrarily low magnetic field. Thermal fluctuations move the magnetization out of the direction of the external field. To maintain the magnetization in the direction of the external field H, the magnetic energy of the particle must be on the order of the thermal energy. Therefore

$$HVM_s\mu_0 \gtrsim k_B T$$

has to be fulfilled in order to be in saturation. Here V is the particle volume, M_s the saturation magnetization of the particles material, k_B the Boltzmann constant, and T the absolute temperature. So, for saturation at low H, the particle volume must be large.

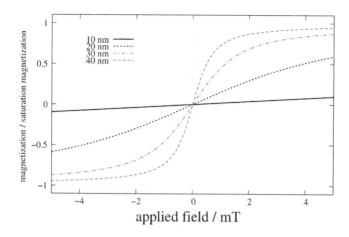

applied field / mT

Figure 4.2: Thermal equilibrium magnetization of spherical magnetite $(0.6\,\mathrm{T}\mu_0^{-1})$ with different diameters at 310 K.

The magnetization curve of small particles in thermal equilibrium is described by the Langevin theory of paramagnetism. The thermodynamic equilibrium magnetization is

$$M = M_0 L \left(\frac{HVM_s\mu_0}{k_{\mathrm{B}}T} \right)$$

with L the Langevin function $L(\alpha) = \coth(\alpha) - \alpha^{-1}$ and M_0 the saturation magnetization of the dispersion of the magnetic particles. Magnetization curves for different magnetite particles sizes at 310 K are plotted in Fig. 4.2.

In the initial explanation of MPI, the feed needed to "saturate" the magnetic material is essential for determining the resolution. For this saturation, a reasonable value has to be found. It is useful to look at the signal induced when a linearly rising external field is applied. When the magnetic material is still very close to the saturation, e.g., at $0.9M_0$, the induced signal is very low compared to the maximum value. So for MPI, a much lower value for the "saturation" has to be chosen. It is reasonable to choose $0.5M_0$ as saturation. Between $-0.5M_0$ and $0.5M_0$, there lies 50 % of the integrated signal. This is similar to a "full width of half maximum" definition of a peak width. Using the Langevin theory, the $0.5M_0$ saturation value for different particle sizes is

Diameter	saturation field	resolution at $3\,\mathrm{T}\mu_0^{-1}/\mathrm{m}$
10 nm	$31\,\mathrm{mT}\mu_0^{-1}$	21 mm
15 nm	$9.1\,\mathrm{mT}\mu_0^{-1}$	6.1 mm
20 nm	$3.8\,\mathrm{mT}\mu_0^{-1}$	2.5 mm
25 nm	$2.0\,\mathrm{mT}\mu_0^{-1}$	1.3 mm
30 nm	$1.1\,\mathrm{mT}\mu_0^{-1}$	0.7 mm
35 nm	$0.72\,\mathrm{mT}\mu_0^{-1}$	0.5 mm
40 nm	$0.48\,\mathrm{mT}\mu_0^{-1}$	0.3 mm

A value of $31\,\mathrm{mT}\mu_0^{-1}$ corresponds to a resolution of 62 mm at a selection field strength of $1\,\mathrm{T}\mu_0^{-1}/\mathrm{m}$, which is probably not enough for
medical imaging. For selection fields of $\leq 3\,\mathrm{T}\mu_0^{-1}/\mathrm{m}$, particles need to
be larger than 20 nm to serve as useful contrast agents for MPI, be-
cause in this constellation the resolution would be only 2.5 to 5 mm[1].
Larger particles increase the resolution and/or reduce the effort needed
to realize a scanner.

4.3 Remagnetization processes

In the previous section, the magnetization curve in thermal equilibrium
was explained. Here it will be explored by which processes this equilibrium can be approached and how fast these processes are. There are
two main mechanisms for the change of magnetization. The first one
is the geometric rotation of the single-domain particle. This process
is often called "Brownian rotation". The second process is the rotation of the magnetization direction itself, i.e., without the rotation of
the crystal. This is called "Neel rotation". Both happen either due
to thermal fluctuations or due to the applied magnetic field. For an
initial magnetization speed discussion, mainly the latter effect must be
discussed.

The speed of the Brownian rotation is determined by the (hydrodynamic) shape of the particle, its average magnetization, and the viscosity of the medium. For a simple estimation of the rotation speed, we

---

[1]The higher value relates to those directions where the selection field gradient strength is only
half of the favoured direction.

assume a cylindrical particle with equal diameter D and length $L = D$. This cylinder is encapsulated in a second cylinder with double the diameter. The viscosity of the medium between the surfaces is η. When ignoring the curvature and effects at the ends of the cylinders, the force due to the viscosity is

$$F = v\eta \frac{\pi DL}{D} = v\eta\pi D$$

where v is the speed at the surface of the inner cylinder. Replacing v by the angular rotation frequency ω we get:

$$F = \frac{\pi}{2}\omega\eta D^2$$

Therefore, the torque on the particle is

$$T = \frac{\pi}{4}\omega\eta D^3$$

This torque has to be balanced by the magnetic torque which is at maximum:

$$T = \frac{MVH}{\mu_0} = \frac{\pi D^3}{4\mu_0}MH$$

Here M is the magnetization of the material, H the external magnetic field and V the cylinder's volume, which can be expressed in terms of D. Combining the two equations and solving for ω we get:

$$\omega = \frac{\mu_0 MH}{\eta}$$

So the rotation speed is independent of the size of the particle. Setting M and H to $1\,\mathrm{T}\mu_0^{-1}$ and η to $1\,\mathrm{mPa\,s}$, which is approximately the viscosity of water, the rotation speed is $\omega \approx 2\pi{\cdot}100\,\mathrm{MHz}$.

In MPI, fields on the order of $1\,\mathrm{mT}\mu_0^{-1}$ are applied. An average magnetization of $1\,\mathrm{T}\mu_0^{-1}$ is already a high value for a magnetic particle and therefore no relevant frequency components above $100\,\mathrm{kHz}$ are expected to emerge from the Brownian magnetization process. An MPI measurement relying on the Brownian rotation would need a drive field frequency much lower than this, e.g., $1\,\mathrm{kHz}$, reducing the encoding speed. For many applications the speed might still be sufficient. The more severe problem is the difficulty of efficiently detecting the signals at these frequencies, which is discussed later.

The Neel rotation can be much faster than the Brownian rotation as it relies on the coherent rotation of the coupled electron spins in the ferromagnet. The maximum speed of the magnetization change is reached when the spin system is critically damped. In this case, the time needed for magnetization reversal is on the order of the reciprocal Larmor frequency. The gyromagnetic ratio of electrons is $28\,\text{GHz}/\text{T}$ which means a maximum generated frequency of $28\,\text{MHz}$ at $1\,\text{mT}\mu_0^{-1}$, which is fast enough for MPI operation.

4.4 Magnetic anisotropy

Looking at the literature on the magnetization of small particles one frequently finds that the Brownian process is called the fast process and the Neel process the slow one. This contradicts the conclusion of the previous section. But it turns out that both statements are correct, depending on the experimental set-up. If you magnetize a suspension of small particles and switch off the magnetic field, the fluid will rapidly lose its magnetization as the orientation of the fine particles will diffuse and assume a random orientation. There is no energy barrier that must be overcome in the Brownian rotation.

If the orientation of the particles is fixed, only Neel rotation can result in a loss of magnetization. But here, energy barriers may exist and the process of losing the magnetization may be slow if the energy barrier considerably exceeds the thermal energy. The existence of high energy barriers allows the use of magnetized particles in data storage, e.g., magnetic tapes and hard disks.

There are three main reasons for energy barriers or anisotropy in magnetic particles. The first one is the so called crystal anisotropy (Fig. 4.3, right). It results from the different potential energies in different magnetization directions relative to the crystal lattice. The second source of energy barriers is the shape anisotropy (Fig. 4.3, left). It is somewhat similar to the demagnetization factor. For a single domain particle it is energetically more favourable to be magnetized in the direction of the largest elongation. The third reason is the so called induced anisotropy. It is an anisotropy that occurs if the magnetic material is mechanically stressed. In a suspensions of small particles, as used in MPI, it does not play an important role.

The anisotropy of the particles has not only an influence on the

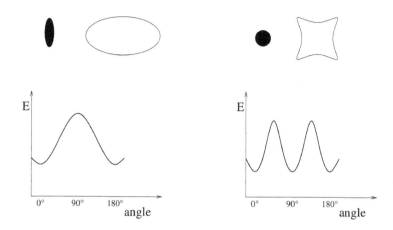

Figure 4.3: The energy landscape of uniaxial (e.g., shape anisotropy, left) and cubic crystal anisotropy. In the upper left, a particle elongated in the top–bottom direction is displayed. Right of the particle, the magnetic energy is sketched in polar coordinates. The magnetic energy is highest if the magnetic vector is oriented horizontally. Therefore the energy landscape is an oblate ellipse. In the bottom of the left part, the energy is plotted against the angle. In the right, the energy landscape of a spherical particle (no shape anisotropy) with cubic lattice symmetry is plotted (cross section). The energy-landscape is no longer uniaxial and more directions of preferred magnetization orientation exist .

speed of reaching thermal equilibrium. It also changes the shape of the magnetization curve as seen in Fig. 4.4. Here a particle with an uniaxial anisotropy is assumed. There is one direction in which the magnetization is preferred (easy axis). The other directions are equivalent to each other. In the left, it is assumed that the easy axis of the particle is parallel to the external magnetic field. In the right, the easy axis is perpendicular to the field. The magnetization curves drawn below the particles show the response of a single particle during one field cycle. In the parallel configuration, the magnetization stays in the original orientation until the strength of the external magnetic field is sufficiently strong to overcome the energy barrier. At this point,

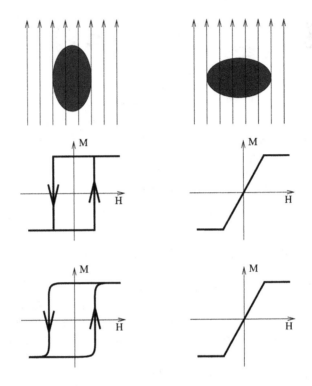

Figure 4.4: The magnetization curves of uniaxial anisotropic particles
and ensembles of anisotropic particles with the easy axis
parallel and perpendicular to the easy axis.

the magnetization suddenly jumps to the opposite direction.

In the case of the orthogonal orientation of the easy axis, the magnetization curve is smooth. At high external fields, the magnetization
is forced into the direction of the field. When the strength is lowered,
the orientation of the magnetization more and more approaches the
direction of the easy axis which is perpendicular to the applied field.
The magnetization in the direction of the external field becomes zero.
Likewise, external magnetic fields can only gradually move the magnetization direction towards the direction of the external field. So the
steepness of the magnetization curve in the parallel case is much higher

than in the orthogonal case. For MPI, this means that in the parallel case, the MPI resolution is much higher than in the orthogonal case.

In the last row of Fig. 4.4, the magnetization curves of ensembles of identical particles are sketched. In the perpendicular case, there is almost no change as the system is always near thermal equilibrium. In the parallel case, the magnetization curve gets smoother. The reason for this is that not all particles change their magnetization simultaneously. Some overcome the barrier earlier than others, because the random thermal fluctuations are higher. So, some particles flip when the remaining barrier height is still several $k_\mathrm{B}T$, most, when the barrier approaches a few $k_\mathrm{B}T$. The rest of the particles flip when the barrier height reaches zero. The consequence for MPI is that the resolution does not rise to infinity. Nevertheless, in the presence of an anisotropy, some resolution improvements might be expected. The anisotropy will also be important for the signal encoding, as discussed later.

4.5 Particle–particle interactions

A further complication in the magnetization process of fine particles is the magnetic particle–particle interaction. There are two main reasons why particle–particle interactions are of importance. First, the attractive forces between particles may result in clustering. Second, clustering (independent of the cause) results in a change of the magnetization curve of the material, which may be a benefit or limit for the MPI performance.

To explore clustering behaviour, we assume a suspension, where the particles freely diffuse. So particles will eventually touch each other and complete clustering is only avoided if clusters can break up by thermal fluctuations. Assuming perfect spherical particles of magnetization M and radius r, the magnetic field on the magnetic axis is [Kne90]

$$H(d) = \frac{m}{2\pi d^3}$$

with $m = \frac{4}{3}\pi r^3 M$ the magnetic dipole moment of the particle. In the limit where a second magnetic particle can be approximated by concentrating its dipole moment to its center, the magnetic energy is:

$$E(d) = \frac{m^2 \mu_0}{2\pi d^3} = \frac{8\mu_0 r^6 \pi M^2}{9d^3} \overset{!}{=} x k_B T$$

The last equality follows from the requirement that the magnetic energy must not exceed x times the thermal energy. x depends on the concentration of the magnetic particles but is usually between 5 and 15, so we can assume 10 for this estimate. For magnetite particles ($M = 0.6$ T) of 40 nm diameter, the allowed distance is roughly 100 nm. This means, the particles with a magnetic core diameter of 40 nm need a shell to reach a total diameter of 100 nm. The shell can be a physical coating, but also, or in addition, a repulsive electrostatic force. As the needed minimum distance of the particles increases with r^2 there is a practical upper limit of a stable suspension somewhere in the range between 40 nm and 100 nm. A way to increase this limit could be suitable alternating magnetic fields applied to the suspension [GW04a] that can be viewed as increasing the temperature in the spin system.

The second aspect to explore is the impact of agglomeration. In general, the behaviour of agglomerated particles can be very complex. So, only some limits can be explored. The first one is an agglomeration of many particles each having a very low intrinsic anisotropy. Then the agglomerated substance behaves like a multi-domain magnetic material which is governed by the demagnetization factor. This means the average magnetic field at an individual single-domain particle is reduced and the magnetization curve becomes less steep. So it is expected that an agglomeration degrades the performance with respect to MPI.

On the other hand, one can have a look at two close by nano-particles in thermal equilibrium. Assuming particles without anisotropy, the particles will orient in a way that both magnetizations point in the direction of the distance vector of the particles, having the same orientation. With the particles being close enough together, the coupling can be strong compared to the thermal energy and both particles act effectively as a single particle with doubled magnetization. So in thermal equilibrium, the magnetization curve is significantly steeper.

As a result, agglomeration of particles can result in a better or worse MPI performance, but it definitely alters the magnetization curve, so forming or breaking of clusters may serve as a contrast mechanism [Gle04b].

5 The Focus Field

In principle, MPI only needs a selection field, a drive field and some receive means. But it turns out that an additional field is needed for physiological and technical reasons.

5.1 Patient safety

Before discussing the imaging properties of MPI it is necessary to briefly introduce some physiological and technical limitations for the applicable field strengths. The most severe limitations exist for the drive field strength and frequency. There are two physiological effects that affect the patient. The first is the nerve stimulation and the second is heating. In the frequency range of 20 kHz to 200 kHz little is known about nerve stimulation. The most reliable value is known from hyperthermia experiments at 100 kHz [WGJ$^+$06], where heating dominates as nothing is reported about nerve stimulation. Maybe at lower frequencies, nerve stimulation would occur before severe heating effects appear. For heating, it is relatively simple to generate a physical model. For a given field distribution the induced voltage is proportional to the frequency f and the field strength H. Therefore the proportionality of the heating power P is given by:

$$P \sim \sigma f^2 H^2,$$

where σ is the conductivity of the tissue. For a frequency dependent $\sigma(f)$, the formula above assumes that the relative change is similar enough in all tissues to keep the current distribution constant. Frequency dependent tissue conductivities can be found in [GLG96]. From this it can be seen that the variations in the conductivity are small in the relevant frequency range.

In the hyperthermia paper [WGJ$^+$06], a field of more than $7 \, \mathrm{mT} \mu_0^{-1}$ at 100 kHz was reported to be tolerable to adult humans in the region of the chest in continuous mode. For shorter periods of time, the applicable field strength can be higher. Additionally, the fields applied in this study were quite homogeneous. By using small coils near the patient's skin, the fields may be produced in a smaller fraction of the patient, thus decreasing the heating and nerve stimulation effect, as smaller current loops are generated.

5.2 Technical limitations

The second reason why a drive field can not reach fields much above the physiological limits is that the dissipation in the coil would become simply too high. This is a consequence of the eddy currents in the drive field coil. For generating large magnetic fields, a coil should contain as much conducting material as possible, i.e., it should be a large and densely filled coil. To counter the skin effect, the conductor must consist of many filaments. But the magnetic field generates eddy currents in the filaments and this generates losses. The more conductors, the more losses. To achieve a reasonably low coil heating, the filaments must be very fine, so high frequency litz wire[1] must be used. Currently, the diameter of the filament in litz wire is limited to about $20\,\mu$m due to the technical processes used by the cable manufacturing companies.

5.3 Additional fields, the focus fields

If the drive field is limited to about $20\,\mathrm{mT}\mu_0^{-1}$ at 25 kHz, the field of view (FOV) would be too small for medical applications to a human. For a selection field of $2\,\mathrm{T}\mu_0^{-1}/\mathrm{m}$ the FOV would be roughly $2 \times 4 \times 4\,\mathrm{cm}^3$. So there is a need for a mechanism to increase the FOV.

One solution is to introduce one more set of orthogonal homogeneous fields called "focus fields". Homogeneous fields move the field free point. These fields need to be quite strong, i.e., about 200 to $300\,\mathrm{mT}\mu_0^{-1}$. To be within the physiological limits, the field may not be altered faster than about $40\,\mathrm{T}\mu_0^{-1}/\mathrm{s}$. This means that the frequency for a full swing is below 50 Hz. The energy stored in the field may be on the order of 30 kJ for a human size system. To reach the physiological limits, a reactive power of more than 6 MW would be needed. For comparison, the reactive power of current MRI gradient systems is from 300 kW to

---

[1]Litz wire is a braded and woven wire made from many individually insulated copper wires

2 MW per axis[2]. So with this technology, the full swing frequency can reach more than 5 Hz.

Using the focus field, the FOV is not expanded, but can be assembled out of small cubes, ellipsoids or other shapes. This results in a high flexibility of the acquisition process. For example, with the focus field, it is possible to selectively image only the surface of the heart, if the coronary arteries will be imaged.

The focus field sequence may also be integrated with the drive field sequence. If, e.g., a Lissajous trajectory with low density is applied via the drive fields, a slight movement via the focus field of the trajectory results in a dense sampling of the space. The focus field can also be used to realize Cartesian sampling, i.e., scanning the object line by line.

---

[2]Reactive power at matched voltage/current conditions. The useful power is typically half of this as the matching conditions change during the field sweep.

6 Resolution, sensitivity and speed

6.1 Unlimited resolution?

A first rough estimate for the resolution was given in the chapter about the Langevin theory of paramagnetism as well as in [GW05]. There, the full width of half maximum of a signal was defined as the resolution. But there might be a better way to define it. For a better insight it is useful to consider a simple one-dimensional imaging process, for example 1D optical microscopy.

In Fig. 6.1 the imaging process is sketched. It is assumed that a detector continuously records the signal intensity S while scanning the object intensity I along the spatial coordinate x. In the first row, the imaging process of a point-like source is sketched. However, the detector receives a signal not only if it is directly above the point source, but also if it is placed next to the source. The point source is spread with an intensity distribution of $P(x - x_0)$, constituting the point spread function with x_0 being the position of the source.

In the middle row of Fig. 6.1, the object has a continuous intensity distribution. Nevertheless, the recorded signal can be predicted if one assumes that the object consists of many (infinite) point sources. Thus, the signal intensity S can be written as a convolution:

$$S(x) = \int\limits_{-\infty}^{\infty} I(x')P(x' - x)\,\mathrm{d}x'$$

In a more elegant way, the convolution can be written in Fourier space as a simple product:

$$\hat{S}(k) = \hat{I}(k)\hat{P}(k)$$

Here, the carets (hats) denote a Fourier transform and k is the transformed x-coordinate.

In the last row of Fig. 6.1, the reconstruction process starting from the measured signal S is sketched. The ultimate goal of imaging is

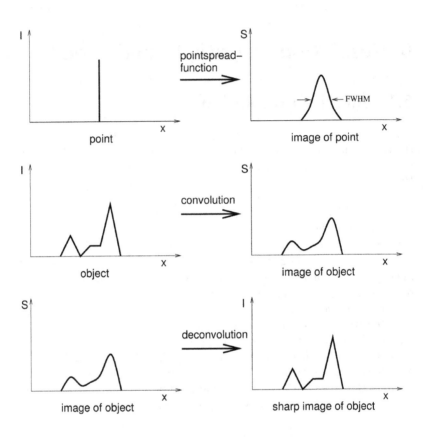

Figure 6.1: Generalized one-dimensional imaging and reconstruction process.

to determine the original intensity distribution I. This can be easily achieved if the equation above is solved for $\hat{I}$:

$$\hat{I}(k) = \frac{\hat{S}(k)}{\hat{P}(k)}$$

So it is possible to compute the image from the measured signal with infinite resolution.[1] The reason why the resolution is not infinite in an actual experiment is the noise. It is not possible to know both S and P with infinite accuracy. The signal intensity in high k-values decreases for both quantities, so it becomes difficult to measure them accurately. The drop is usually significant for k-values that correspond to the full width of half maximum (FWHM) of the point spread function. Therefore using the width of the point spread function as a measure of the resolution seems to be justified. Nevertheless, without knowing the signal to noise ratio (SNR), it is impossible to predict the resolution.

The FWHM of the point spread function can be determined using the magnetization curve and the strength of the selection field gradient. The induced voltage (i.e., the signal strength) is proportional to the derivative of the magnetization curve. Let X_s be the difference in the applied field between the maximum of the derivative and where it reaches half of this maximum. Then the full width of half maximum is:

$$\text{FWHM} = \frac{2X_s}{G}$$

with G being the gradient strength of the selection field.

Maxwell's equations do not allow a field free point with a uniform derivative of the field magnitude in all spatial directions. Instead there is one preferred direction with higher gradient strength. The derivative has its minima in the perpendicular directions and reaches only half of the maximum value. So the resolution in MPI is intrinsically anisotropic.

6.2 Sensitivity

The ability of MPI to detect magnetic material is ultimately limited by the signal to noise ratio (SNR). To determine the sensitivity of MPI,

---

[1]Zeros in $\hat{P}(k)$ are no problem in this ideal version as $\hat{S}(k)$ is zero as well.

it is necessary to know both the optimal induced signal and the lowest possible noise.

6.2.1 Signal strength

For the determination of the signal strength, it is useful to assume that in a volume V the total magnetization m oscillates with an angular frequency of ω. The induced voltage in a recording coil therefore is:

$$U_{\text{ind}}(t) = s\,\omega\,m\,V\cos(\omega t)$$

where s is the sensitivity of the coil defined as the magnetic induction produced at the position of the magnetization divided by the current through the coil. Due to the reciprocity of an antenna, it also connects the induced voltage with the change of magnetization.

In an MPI experiment, the magnetization does not change harmonically and the induced voltage at the base frequency is not recorded. Nevertheless, this approximation seems to be justified. If the magnetic material were to reach saturation instantaneously, the signal amplitude of the third harmonics would still be $\frac{4}{3\pi} \approx 0.42$ of the maximum value.

6.2.2 Patient noise

The lowest possible noise for the detection of magnetic material can be achieved if the instrumentation does not contribute any noise. In this case, the total noise is not zero, as the measured object—the patient—still generates some noise. In the case of examining human tissue, the dominating noise source is the random thermal current fluctuations in the conducting tissue. For the quantification of this noise it is useful to use the fluctuation dissipation theorem [Cal85]. An alternating current in a coil near the patient generates an oscillating magnetic field in the patient. This magnetic field is associated with an electrical field inducing a current in the patient. The finite resistance of the patient leads to a dissipation. The dissipation must result in a real part of the resistance R of the coil and thus the noise voltage is given by:

$$U_n = \sqrt{4k_B T R \Delta f}$$

Here, T is the absolute temperature, k_B Boltzmann's constant, and Δf the frequency band width.

The frequency dependence of the patient noise, i.e., R, is of importance. At a given current through the coil, the induced current in the patient is proportional to the frequency ω. This assumes that the resistivity of the patient is constant over frequency, which although not entirely true, is almost true [Rös87]. The dissipation is proportional to the square of the induced current and therefore proportional to ω^2. Likewise,

$$R \sim \omega^2$$

and

$$U_n \sim \omega$$

As a result, the noise voltage is proportional to the frequency. In the previous section, it was found that the signal voltage is proportional to the frequency used. So, in principle, the ultimate signal to noise ratio is independent of the drive field frequency used.

6.2.3 Detection limit of MPI

For the determination of the absolute value of the detection limit, a specific coil and patient has to be assumed. For simplicity, a coil with a square shape and and a side length of 10 cm will be assumed. The sample is placed in a distance of 10 cm from the center of the coil. Using the law of Biot-Savart the sensitivity of the coil at this point is about $1 \cdot 10^{-6} \frac{T}{A}$. The increase of the resistance of such a coil when placed at the chest of an adult human measured at 20 MHz is roughly 100 mΩ. 1 pg of iron oxide has a dipole moment 92 fAm^2. At 20 MHz this induces a voltage of 12 pV amplitude or 8 pV root mean square (rms). The noise voltage of 100 mΩ is 40 pV/$\sqrt{Hz}$ rms. Assuming that the signal must be 5 times the noise for a reliable detection, one needs roughly 25 pg iron oxide to be able to detect it within 1 second in a human. As the detection limit goes down with the reciprocal square root of the measuring time, 1 pg of iron oxide can be detected within 625 seconds which is roughly 10 minutes.

In the medical community, amounts of iron oxide are specified in Mol of iron atoms. There are 13 mmol(Fe) in 1 g of Fe_3O_4. Therefore the 1 pg detection limit is about 13 fmol of iron.

It is also common to state the detection limit as a concentration. As a consequence, the amount of magnetic material has to be diluted in a voxel. Assuming a voxel size of $1\,\mathrm{mm}^3$, the detectable local concentration is $13\,\mathrm{nmol(Fe)/l}$. For voxel of a size of $1\,\mathrm{cm}^3$, the detection limit is $13\,\mathrm{pmol(Fe)/l}$.

6.2.4 Detection limit of MRI

To give these numbers meaning, they have to be compared to other imaging modalities. The detection limit of magnetic resonance imaging depends in a complicated way on the experimental setting. In small animals and in samples with low background variation, it is quite easy to detect a single cell loaded with a few pg of iron oxide [SGB+06]. The detection of such a low quantity of iron relies on the fact that the susceptibility artifact of the single cell can be seen. But with the currently achievable resolution in a human it is impossible to detect such an artifact. Therefore one has to stick to measuring the change in the relaxation times, especially in T_2 and T_2^* to detect the magnetic material. Here, a lower limit is given by the underlying natural variation in the relaxation rates. This limits the sensitivity to roughly $50\,\mu\mathrm{mol(Fe)/l}$ largely independent of the voxel size.

6.2.5 Detection limit of CT

In CT, the detection of a tracer is limited by the photon statistics and also by the natural variations in tissues. The photon statistics is relatively easy to compute. To keep the calculation simple, it is assumed that all X-ray energy is applied in a single projection. If the dosage is distributed over several projections, like in CT, the sensitivity can not be better. This can be seen, if a rotational symmetric object is examined with the additional absorber in the middle. In this situation, all the projections can be combined into one projection without gain or loss of information. The limiting factor is the allowed average tissue dosage. The dosage d (unit: energy/volume) may reach locally $100\,\mathrm{mJ/l}$. For CT, $20\,\mathrm{mJ/kg}$ i.e., about $20\,\mathrm{mJ/kg}$ of body mass is already a high dose, but usually, only a fraction of the body is scanned. The ray penetrates a length l (assumed to be $0.4\,\mathrm{m}$) of the body and the photons are counted on the other side. If the linear dimension (side length) of a voxel is v, the incident X-ray energy on the surface of the body through th voxel is:

$$E_i = dlv^2$$

The body tissue absorbs or scatters most of this energy. The energy at the detector is

$$E_d = E_i e^{-\mu l} = dlv^2 e^{-\mu l}$$

The attenuation coefficient μ is about $10\,\mathrm{m}^{-1}$ for p=50 keV photon energy. The number of photons at the detector is

$$N = \frac{E_d}{p} = \frac{dlv^2}{p} e^{-\mu l}$$

If an additional absorber is brought into the ray, the number of photons will decrease by ΔN. This number can be derived from the mass attenuation coefficient μ_m, the molar mass M, the molar concentration c and the absorber length, which is in our case v:

$$\Delta N = N(1 - e^{\mu_m M c v}) \approx N \mu_m M c v$$

For low relative changes of the photon number, the approximation is valid. To reliably detect the additional absorber, a change of five times the noise level may be assumed, therefore,

$$\Delta N = 5\sqrt{N}$$

$$\frac{dlv^2}{p} e^{-\mu l} \mu_m M c v = 5\sqrt{\frac{dlv^2}{p} e^{-\mu l}}$$

This has to be solved to achieve the minimal detectable concentration c:

$$c = \frac{5}{\mu_m M v^2} \sqrt{\frac{p}{dl} e^{\mu l}}$$

For gadolinium (M =157 g/mol), the mass attenuation coefficient is 18.6 cm^2/g at 50.2 keV, i.e., right above the K-edge. Therefore, the 1 mm^3 detection limit is

$$c_{\mathrm{Gd}} \approx 1.8\,\mathrm{mmol/l}$$

For bismuth (M =209 g/mol), the mass attenuation coefficient is 84 cm^2/g. Therefore the detection limit is somewhat lower:

$$c_{\mathrm{Bi}} \approx 0.3\,\mathrm{mmol/l}$$

The estimates above assumed that the initial absorption (without contrast agent) is known with infinite accuracy and without any additional

X-ray dose. In reality, there is noise and additional dose regardless of whether a reference scan without tracer is performed or the K-edge is used for a virtual tracer free image. Therefore the real detection limits are higher by a factor of 2 for the given X-ray dose. An additional effect is that a conventional X-ray tube produces a broad spectrum with many sub-optimal photon energies. This increases the detection limit further. So it is safe to assume that CT detection limits lie above 1 mmol/l. Even for a 5 mm linear voxel size, the gadolinium detection limit will be higher than 150 μmol/l. A CT sensitivity analysis for energy resolved detectors (K-edge imaging) can be found in [RBS+08].

6.2.6 Detection limit of PET and SPECT

Nuclear methods are much more sensitive than MPI. In PET about 1% of the annihilations can be recorded. Assuming 100 counts for a minimum detection, a total of 10^4 disintegrations are needed. A typical measuring time of 1000 seconds may be assumed, so 10 Bq is the minimum activity one can detect in one voxel. For ^{18}F, 10^5 atoms, i.e., $2 \cdot 10^{-19}$ mol, are needed to generate 10 decays per second. For 1 mm^3 voxel, this would be a concentration of 0.2 pmol/l, but such high resolutions are not feasible for clinical PET scanners. A resolution of 5 mm is more realistic and therefore a detection limit of 2 fmol/l. For this, the total applied dosage for a 75 kg human would be 600 kBq. In clinical applications much more dosage is applied, typically 300 MBq, as in most cases the contrast between healthy and diseased tissue is small. Uptake increase in tumors is often less than double than in healthy tissue [MTO+08].

SPECT has roughly 1% sensitivity of PET, as most of the photons are absorbed in the collimator. Nevertheless sensitivity is still high compared to MPI sensitivity.

In conclusion, MPI has a high sensitivity considerably exceeding the sensitivity of CT and MRI. Nevertheless, the nuclear methods are much more sensitive than MPI. Still there are advantages of MPI over the nuclear methods.

In applications where ultimate sensitivity is not needed (e.g., perfusion and lung ventilation), MPI has the advantage of of using a tracer with a long shelf-life and of not using ionizing radiation.

In applications with a need for high sensitivity, but a slow physiological mechanism of enrichment (e.g., cell tracking), MPI may exceed the nuclear methods in terms of sensitivity. The reason is that the particles do not decay rapidly[2]. So at measurement time, the original amount of magnetic particles is still present, but commonly used radiopharmaceuticals (^{99m}Tc) have decayed to a very small concentration.

6.3 Encoding efficiency

A detection limit of roughly 1 pg of iron oxide was determined in the previous section, using the signal emission from a single voxel. If MPI were to be used in the way initially described in [GW05], i.e., with a modulation field, only one voxel at a time would generate a signal. If one wants to measure N voxels to generate a complete image, one would need N times the time needed for a single voxel. Alternatively, if keeping the measuring time constant, the detection limit increases by $\sqrt{N}$ as it is proportional to the inverse square root of the measuring time. A medical image typically contains 256×256 voxels or more. So the detection limit for a 10 minute acquisition time would be reduced to 256 pg per voxel or 3.3 μmol/l for 1 mm^3 voxel. This might not be good enough to justify the development of a new imaging method. So there is a need for an encoding that is more efficient than the single voxel method.

Magnetic resonance imaging (MRI) had a similar problem. The magnetic dipole moment of the protons in one cubic millimeter of water is 6 pAm^2 at 1 Tμ_0^{-1} external field. This is equivalent to roughly 70 pg of iron oxide. If one would acquire an MRI image voxel by voxel, as initially proposed in [Dam72], high resolution imaging would be impossible.

In MRI, frequency and phase encoding helped to solve the sensitivity problem. The basic principle is to acquire information from many voxels simultaneously. The frequency encoding (Fig. 6.2, upper left part) is the encoding mechanism which is easiest to understand. We assume that all voxels lie on a line. If a gradient field is applied, all voxels along the line get their own frequency. So it is possible to measure all voxels simultaneously. The noise bandwidth per voxel is still the

---

[2]Blood clearance is usually fast, but intracellular decay time constants vary from days to month depending on the type of coating

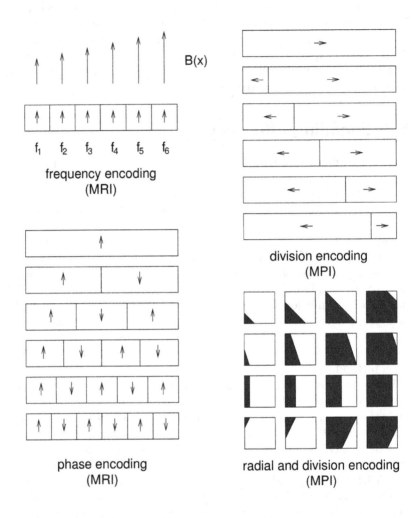

Figure 6.2: Encoding mechanisms in magnetic resonance imaging (MRI) and MPI. Two regions of magnetization in opposite directions are separated by a moving and rotation line/plane.

inverse of the measuring time, so in the frequency encoded images, all voxels have a quality as if each voxel was measured the total measuring time individually.

Phase encoding (Fig. 6.2, lower left part) uses different sums and differences of signals in a way that the individual response of a single voxel can be computed. It turns out that this encoding mechanism is as good as the frequency encoding in terms of signal to noise ratio.

So, for MPI it is also necessary to acquire a signal from many voxels simultaneously. Introducing a drive field, i.e., quickly moving the field free point a distance much longer than a voxel diameter, leads to a sort of simultaneous acquisition as sketched in Fig. 6.2 upper right part. In this "division encoding" the FFP divides two regions. So at a given time, the magnetization left of the FFP minus the magnetization right of the FFP is measured.

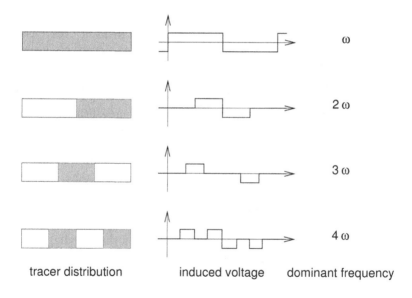

tracer distribution   induced voltage   dominant frequency

Figure 6.3: Induced voltage for spatial distributions mimicking a Fourier series. The dominant harmonics in the induced signal correspond to the spatial Fourier series with an offset of one. So the spatial $0k$ corresponds to 1ω, $1k$ corresponds to 2ω and so on.

This encoding can be viewed as a phase encoding in the frequency domain. Assume that the magnetic material is homogeneously distributed over the entire line. Then the magnetization is proportional to the position of the FFP and therefore (almost) proportional to the drive field. So the signal of the integral of the concentration is mainly in the fundamental frequency ω of the drive field. If the magnetic material is mainly in the left part, a dominant signal is generated at 2ω. Magnetic material present in the middle of three equal sections produces mainly a signal at 3ω and so on (see Fig. 6.3). So each harmonic contains the corresponding spatial Fourier transform of the material concentration. If a triangular drive field is introduced, this becomes exactly true. Assuming ideal particles, the signal amplitude for the ideal particle is identical for all harmonics. This can be seen by assuming a Dirac δ like particle concentration (i.e., a spot of tracer without any physical extend, but a finite amount or particles) that produces a step function in the magnetization and therefore a δ spike in the induced voltage. The Fourier transform of a δ distribution is a flat frequency response.

Now one could assume that the encoding efficiency in a one-dimensional MPI experiment is even better than phase encoding in MRI. In phase encoding, one needs N steps to acquire the spatial Fourier transforms, but in MPI, all information is acquired simultaneously. So the encoding should be a factor $\sqrt{N}$ more efficient in terms of SNR. Unfortunately, this is not the case for a patient-noise limited recording system. Here the noise floor amplitude rises proportionally to the frequency. So at the highest spatial frequency, corresponding to $N\omega$, the SNR is a factor $\sqrt{N}$ lower than in phase encoding. On the other hand, the presence of magnetic material (low resolution) can be measured much more accurately than in the phase encoding approach.

The "division encoding" in one dimension has some properties that are better and some properties that are worse than the encodings used in MRI. For encodings in two or three dimensions it is in principle possible to use encoding schemes known from MRI and CT. This has been elaborated in [WGB08]. It is possible to create a field free line instead of a field free point. If the line scans over the object, a signal is produced along the whole line. For encoding an image, the line has to be turned as shown in Fig. 6.2 (lower right). This encoding is equivalent to a radial sequence in MRI, which is known to be similarly efficient as the phase encoding step.

However, the field free line for 2D encoding can not be generalized to a "field free plane" in 3D. The reason is that Maxwell's equations do not allow a field free plane in a source free region, neglecting the trivial solution of a completely field free space. So for an efficient 3D encoding a different mechanism has to be found.

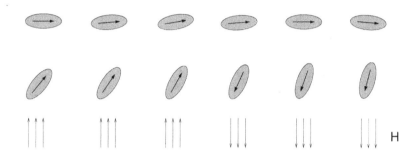

Figure 6.4: Behaviour of an anisotropic particle in an oscillating magnetic field. In the top row, the particles' easy axis is aligned approximately perpendicularly to the oscillating magnetic field. The torque on the particle during the field's "up" period is exactly canceled by the torque in the "down" period. In the lower row, the particle is already to some degree aligned to the external field direction.

It may be possible to construct an emulation for field free plane using the anisotropy of the magnetic particles ("virtual field free plane"). This is illustrated in Fig. 6.4. The first ingredient of the virtual field free plane is the tendency of anisotropic particles to align with their easy axis along the direction of the drive field even in the presence of a static magnetic (selection) field. The reason for this is the combination of the Brownian (geometric) rotation and the Neel rotation as illustrated in the figure. Therefore a simple sequence moving an FFP along a line creates a region of aligned particles. The lateral size of the region is roughly equivalent to the distance the FFP moves.

Therefore the magnetization points upwards until a substantial reverse magnetic field is applied. Then the magnetization flips immediately (Fig.6.5). Due to the anisotropy, the particles magnetization

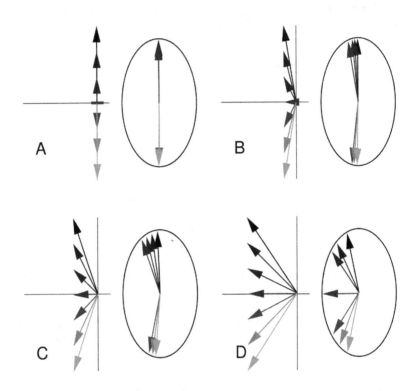

Figure 6.5: Magnetization change in an aligned particle. In the left of the images A, B, C and D, the external magnetic field vector is plotted. The arrows in the ellipses indicate the magnetization directions. The time evolves from dark to brighter arrows, i.e., from arrows pointing to the top to arrows pointing to the bottom. In A, the magnetic field and the easy axis are perfectly aligned. In B, a small, but constant perpendicular field is added.

still points in plus or minus easy axis direction. Only small deviations from the easy axis are observed. These deviations gradually increase when the perpendicular field is increased as in C. But when the perpendicular field reaches the anisotropy field of the particle, like in D, the magnetization vector smoothly follows the external field without a jump.

The second effect needed for a virtual field free plane is the fact that the magnetic particles are mainly sensitive to the field component parallel to the easy axis of the particle (Figs. 4.4 and 6.5). Perpendicular components do not have a significant effect as long as the field strength is insufficient to overcome the barrier height. Then the magnetization stays almost in the direction of the easy axis.

Now if a field in the direction of the easy axis is applied, the barrier is eventually overcome and the magnetization flips. This magnetization flip occurs simultaneously along a plane, or more precisely, a slightly curved surface. So there exists a flat, almost two-dimensional object, where the signal is generated simultaneously. This is what is needed for efficient encoding.

The final step is simple: the plane has to be rotated to fill the Radon space completely (Fig. 6.2, lower right). The conceptually simplest way is to rotate all fields, but this would be a technical challenge. Fortunately it may be not necessary to turn everything, but only the oscillation direction of the field free point, i.e., the field free point trajectory is a rosette.

Experimental evidence that this type of encoding may actually work is given in Fig. 6.6. In a 1D sequence, the lateral extension of the signal generation area is much larger than expected from the simulation. The grey value of each pixel was determined as follows. A small sample (diameter 0.5 mm, length 1 mm) was set to the position corresponding to the pixel position and the drive field was applied. The recorded signal was Fourier transformed and the real part of the Fourier component at 0, f, $2f$ and so on is proportional to the pixel grey value in the corresponding tiles. So one measurement defines the grey value of exactly the same pixel in all tiles. So both the alignment of the particles in the oscillating field and the resulting higher signal to noise ratio are likely to happen in reality. Further evidence for particle alignment is presented in the section "temperature imaging" (9.4).

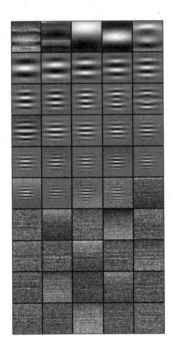 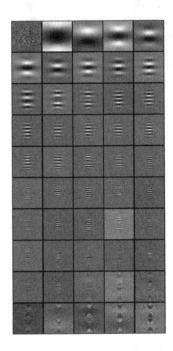

Figure 6.6: Comparison of the spatial response of experimental (left) and simulated (right) particles. The drive field had an amplitude of $10\,\mathrm{mT}\mu_0^{-1}$ at $f{=}25\,\mathrm{kHz}$ in the up–down direction. The selection field strength was about $3\,\mathrm{T}\mu_0^{-1}/\mathrm{m}$ with the strongest gradient also in the up–down direction. Simulation by the Langevin theory. The $5{\times}10$ tiles in each image correspond to one frequency increasing from left-top to right-bottom. The first frequency is 0, the second f the third $2f$ and so on. Each tile consists of $52{\times}52$ pixels, covering an area of about $1{\times}1\,\mathrm{cm}^2$. In the experimental results, the signal is generated from a considerably larger area than in the simulated data.

6.4 Speed limit

In the previous section, mechanisms have been discussed to maintain a good signal to noise ratio when encoding an image. As quite high local concentrations of a tracer material can be reached, for example in a bolus injection, the SNR would allow fast imaging. But this is not enough. Also the encoding has to be fast.

6.4.1 MPI encoding speed

The encoding speed in MPI is determined by the drive field amplitude, the drive field frequency, and the tracer performance. The number of voxels per unit time R that one can record is approximately

$$R_{\text{MPI}} = \frac{4Af}{2X_s} = \frac{2Af}{X_s}$$

This formula can be derived as follows: During one period, i.e., the reciprocal of the frequency f, the field changes four times from zero to the amplitude A or back. Therefore, the total field change is $4A$. By definition, $2X_s$ is the field change needed to encode one voxel, assuming the full with of half maximum (FWHM) definition for the resolution. In the previous section, a link between the resolution and signal to noise ratio was derived. Therefore, the formula above is not valid for all conditions. Nevertheless, it seems to be accurate enough for tracer concentrations in medical imaging.

The drive field amplitude and frequency are limited by the physiological tolerance of the patient as discussed in Section 5.1. In hyperthermia experiments [WGJ+06], it was possible to apply $7\,\text{mT}\mu_0^{-1}$ at $100\,\text{kHz}$ which can be assumed as a lower limit of the field strength frequency product. For X_s one may use the value for $30\,\text{nm}$ ideal (Langevin theory) iron oxide nano-particles of $1.1\,\text{mT}\mu_0^{-1}$. In [GW05] it was shown that Resovist has particles of this size in its composition. Setting the values in the formula above, one can expect at least $R_{\text{MPI}} \approx 1.3$ million voxels per second. Sensitivity encoding, i.e., recording the signal of multiple coils in parallel, may be be a way to raise this value. The signal in MPI is usually recorded by at least three coils (orthogonal directions). The signals from these coils are not identical and contain complementary information about the position of the magnetic material. So the voxel rate may be increased by a factor of 3. Additionally, for short acquisition times, higher fields or frequencies can be applied without heating the patient too much, thus further increasing the voxel rate. Therefore voxel rates exceeding 10 million per second seem to be feasible.

The number of voxels per second has to be related to other imaging modalities. There are two important tasks for this comparison. First, it has to be compared to the physical and physiological limits of the modalities, second, it has be compared to the technical implementations existing today.

6.4.2 Ultrasound encoding speed

The theoretical voxel rate of ultrasound can be estimated as follows: With the voxel size d, the time of encoding one voxel is d/c. Here c is the speed of sound. Assuming $1\,\mathrm{mm}$ voxel size and $c \approx 1500\,\mathrm{m/s}$ for soft tissue [Mor95], the voxel rate is about 1.5 mega-voxel per second. This can be increased by the number of detectors to N. As long as the detectors are not closer to each other than the voxel size, all detectors can contribute equally to the voxel rate. So, the total rate is

$$R_{\mathrm{US}} = \frac{Nc}{d}$$

Theoretically, the number of detectors may be up to 10^5, so 150 giga-voxel per second would be possible. With current technology, the number of independent detectors can still be above 100. So it is feasible that ultrasound reach the giga-voxel per second range, thus clearly exceeding the other imaging modalities. Available products seem to exceed 100 mega-voxel per second.

6.4.3 CT encoding speed

Computed X-ray tomography (CT) can also be parallelized using many detector elements. The speed limit is

$$R_{\mathrm{CT}} = \frac{2NM}{T_{\mathrm{rot}}},$$

where T_{rot} is the rotation time of the gantry, N the number of simultaneously recorded slices, and M the number of detector elements in one slice. In principle, the rotation speed is unlimited. So there is no physical limit for the voxel rate. There is also no physiological limit to the speed. Only the total number of voxels is limited by the tolerable radiation dose.

Practical limitations are the X-ray power, detector speed, and cost. Still the voxel rate in current CT systems is high: For a field of view of $40\times40\,\mathrm{cm}^2$ and linear voxel dimensions of $1\,\mathrm{mm}$, M is $160\cdot10^3$. N is 256 for current systems and the rotation time reaches 0.2 seconds. So, the voxel rate exceeds $200\cdot10^6$ per second and thus is on a par with the practical level of ultrasound.

6.4.4 MRI encoding speed

In magnetic resonance imaging, the recording bandwidth (in Hz) ultimately limits the number of voxels to be recorded per second as the bandwidth limits the acquisition of information. The bandwidth is given by the product of the gyromagnetic ratio γ, the gradient strength G, and the diameter of the field of view D:

$$R_{\mathrm{MRI}} = \gamma G D.$$

For protons, γ is $42\,\mathrm{MHz/T}$. G is typically limited to $40\,\mathrm{mT/m}$ for physiological reasons, because the gradients have to be switched quickly and higher amplitudes may lead to nerve stimulation. The diameter of the FOV is not larger than $40\,\mathrm{cm}$ for a commercial MRI scanner. As a result, the recording rate is somewhat below 700 kilo-voxel per second.

Practically, the voxel rate is usually much lower due to the necessary delays for contrast generation. Other limiting factors can be the time needed to select a sub-volume (slices), or the delays needed to reduce the SAR. Additionally, the maximum gradient is not applied all the time due to the limited rise time. So the practical voxel rate hardly ever exceeds 100 kilo-voxel per second.

MRI may be accelerated by parallel imaging methods like SENSE [PWSB99]. These use signals from several (N) coils to acquire more information per time out of the image. N is usually a small number, e.g., 4, as the sensitivities of the coils have to be significantly different in the coverage of the FOV. So, 100 kilo-voxel per second still holds as a practical maximum.

As a first conclusion, MPI may be one or two orders of magnitude faster than MRI in terms of voxel rate, but is clearly inferior to CT and ultrasound.

Nevertheless, MPI may have some properties that can deliver a speed superior to CT in some applications. The reason for this is that in MPI, a direct encoding of the space is possible. In MRI and CT, it is necessary to acquire at least a full slice containing many voxels. If, for example, only the inflow of a contrast agent into the coronary arteries has to be displayed, the slices contain many unnecessary voxels. To compare the necessary voxels in MPI and CT/MRI, one can assume that the total length of the coronaries to be imaged is 0.5 meter and that one needs to acquire one square centimeter around each coronary. Then the number of $1\,\text{mm}^3$ sized voxels to be recorded is about $5 \cdot 10^4$, i.e., full encoding may be achieved in 5 to 50 milliseconds using MPI. CT and MRI have to encode a volume of roughly $400 \times 300 \times 100\,\text{mm}^3$ containing $12 \cdot 10^6$ voxel, which is 240 times the number of voxels needed in MPI.

7 Experimental and simulation results on MPI

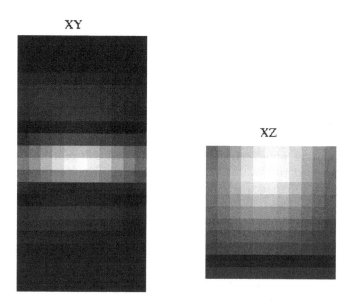

Figure 7.1: The first MPI image acquired in 2001. Each 3D voxel had an isotropic size of 1 mm. The cylindrical phantom had a diameter of 2 mm in the X and Z directions and a length of 3 mm in the Y direction. The left image shows an X–Y slice, containing the voxel of highest intensity. In the right image, an X–Z slice is shown, also containing this voxel.

The first MPI image was acquired in 2001 [1], but never previously published. In Fig. 7.1 two slices of the volume data are presented. The phantom consisted of a tube (2 mm diameter 3 mm length) filled with an iron oxide suspension. The recording coil was directly wound on the phantom and only the magnitude of the third harmonics was recorded using an analogue filter and rectifier. The grey value of the image directly represents this recorded magnitude. The sample was centred in a drive field coil operating at 220 kHz and a field amplitude between 1 and $2\,mT\mu_0^{-1}$. Thus, this measurement very well reflects the "modulation field" approach as described in [GW05]. Two copper coils generated a selection field of strength about $0.5\,T\mu_0^{-1}/m$ with the highest gradient in drive field direction. The sample, recording coil, and drive field coil assembly was moved in the selection field using a robot.

The image shows already a quite good resolution on the order of 3 mm in the Y-direction. But there are two side lobes, typical for the third harmonics response's blurring the image to 1.5 cm in the Y direction. However, the lobes have a relatively low intensity. A reconstruction would help to get rid of these lobes. The resolution in the X–Z direction is about 6 mm, because the selection field strength in this direction is lower.

After several improvements in hardware and software, the image quality reached the level displayed in Fig. 7.2. This result was also published in [GW05], where details about the imaging set-up and sequence can be found. While the image resolution displayed in the images would be good enough for a medical application, the acquisition time of almost one hour was by far too long. Also the concentration of 500 mmol(Fe)/l was at least a factor of 100 too high compared to concentrations expected in clinical applications.

In simulation studies [WBG07] and [WGB08], MPI scanners with dimensions suitable for an adult human have been analysed. The results showed that if all technical difficulties can be overcome, the image quality and speed should be good enough for medical applications.

A massive increase in speed was demonstrated experimentally in [GWB08]. Frames from an image sequence are shown in Fig. 7.3 displaying different acquisition times. One frame was encoded in about 4 ms, resulting in 250 images per second. Again, for a clinical applica-

---

[1]precisely on 2001/5/23

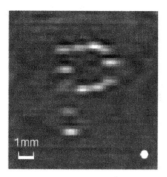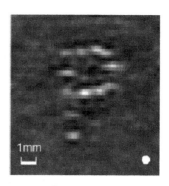

Figure 7.2: Two 2D images published in [GW05]. The dot in the bottom right indicates the true size of the iron oxide filled holes in the phantom. Not all dots in the phantom were properly filled. The image in the left uses all acquired information, while in the right, only a fraction of the robot positions were used. This demonstrates that faster image acquisition would be feasible.

tion, the 500 mmol(Fe)/l concentration was still much too high.

This limitation was finally overcome in [WGR+09], reporting the first 3D *in vivo* results on magnetic particle imaging. Some of the results shown were acquired using an approved Resovist dosage 10 μmol/l. The presented real-time volume (3D) images display a temporal resolution suitable for blood flow evaluation. In addition to the data analysis in the paper, the blood flow velocity in the *vena cava* of a mouse was assessed as seen in Fig. 7.4. A simple tracking of the bolus peak was sufficient and the approximated 6 mm/s speed of blood flow seemed to be realistic for a heavily sedated mouse.

The next steps for bringing MPI to human use should be scaling the scanner hardware to larger sizes while maintaining the image quality. Usually, the image quality degrades when scaling up a scanner. According to [WGR+09], it seems that there is still enough room for improvement in the scanner hardware that the image quality could be maintained in a human size system. In addition, improvements of the contrast agent have potential that images in a clinical system could exceed the mouse images shown in terms of resolution and sensitivity.

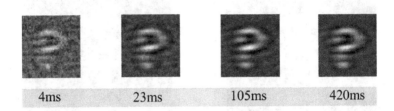

Figure 7.3: Single frames of a video acquisition of a moved phantom published in [GWB08]. The numbers under the images are the integration times for the images, i.e., the time of acquisition.

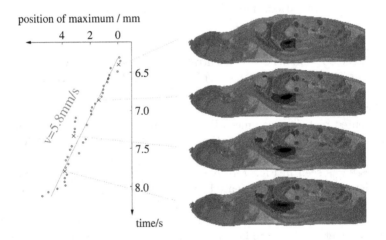

Figure 7.4: Tracer inflow through the *vena cava* of a mouse after bolus injection into the tail vein. The dynamic MPI data (dark colors) are superimposed in the MRI images using a suitable threshold. For details see [WGR+09].

8 Potential applications of MPI

After exploring the basic imaging properties of MPI, potential applications for MPI will then be discussed. With the current status of
knowledge, it is not possible to predict which of the applications will
come to clinical routine use. However, in many areas, improvements
of current procedures seem possible, and as MPI is still in a very early
state, many applications might be possible that are currently out of
clinical reach.

8.1 Combination with magnetic resonance imaging

Before discussing specific applications, it is necessary to discuss scenarios for the provision of an "anatomical reference". MPI images the
distribution of magnetic particles. To interpret these data, it is help-
ful to refer to an image of the underlying anatomy. There are many
ways to get this information. The simplest is to register images of
other modalities to MPI images using markers that can be identified
in both modalities. It is also possible to place a CT system next to an
MPI scanner. When using the same patient support for both modalities (called "shared table"), registration of the images becomes simple.
Nevertheless, some sort of fusion is still necessary, possibly leading to
uncertainties in the fused images. Also, the additional imaging system
involves a higher cost and more effort in patient handling.

Therefore, an intrinsic combination of MPI with an anatomical reference image seems to be useful. One such combination would be with
magnetic resonance imaging which seems to be technically feasible.
Both MPI and MRI use strong magnetic fields and record weak oscillating fields. The field geometries and frequencies are not identical,
but with moderate technical effort components may be designed serv-
ing both MPI and MRI. For example, if the selection field in MPI is

generated by electromagnets, a reverse current in one coil yields a homogeneous field suitable for polarizing the protons. The field strength for MRI may reach $0.5\,\mathrm{T}$ for resistive coils and $1\,\mathrm{T}$ or more for superconducting coils.

There are a variety of effects that make an intrinsic MPI/MRI combination problematic. For MRI, the fields need to be very homogeneous but simply changing the current direction in one coil usually does not provide a field with sufficient homogeneity because such a coil assembly would be not very efficient for selection field generation. The MPI system contains no transmitter for the RF (B_1) field and no recording system for frequencies as high as several tens of MHz. Moreover, the MPI drive and recording coils have self-resonances in the low MHz range making the addition of a MRI B_1 coil difficult.

One solution for these technical challenges would be to construct a field cycling or pre-polarized MRI system [MC93]. In such a system, a strong, but not necessarily very homogeneous, field is applied for several hundred milliseconds to polarize the protons. After the polarizing pulse the field is reduced to a much lower value where the RF pulses are applied. In MRI, the field homogeneity needs to be roughly $10\,\mu\mathrm{T}\mu_0^{-1}$ which is $10\,\mathrm{ppm}$ for a $1\,\mathrm{T}$ scanner but $1\,\%$ for a $1\,\mathrm{mT}$ scanner. Such a value could be reached by changing the current direction in the selection field coils.

Going to such a low field, the RF pulses can be applied using the drive field coil. The Larmor frequency of protons at $0.6\,\mathrm{mT}$ is $25\,\mathrm{kHz}$, i.e., the currently used MPI drive field frequency. The drive field amplitudes in an MPI scanner exceed the necessary amplitudes for MRI by far. An alternative to the drive field for the RF pulse is the focus field. It contains frequency components of up to about $1\,\mathrm{kHz}$. Therefore, the B_0 field has to be even lower, when applying the RF pulse. The focus field amplitude is so high that the RF pulse may be described as:

1. Polarize the protons using a strong B_0.

2. Reduce the field strength to zero.

3. Increase the field value using a direction which is not identical with the proton polarization. This is the "RF pulse", i.e., the cause of precession.

4. Ramp the field up to achieve a convenient Larmor frequency for

signal recording (e.g., 1 MHz) and apply a suitable sequence of gradients.

A spin echo using this method would be a simple field reversal.

A pre-polarized MRI would certainly be sufficient for the anatomical reference in MPI. For some selected applications, it may be even superior to the traditional way of MRI. For patients with implants, a pre-polarized MRI would allow near implant imaging as long as the implant is not ferromagnetic [VMR⁺06]. The MPI/MRI combination would be able to operate at even lower frequencies than used in [VMR⁺06], therefore it would be possible to image inside of metallic stents, possibly assessing re-stenosis.

The field cycling allows contrasts not attainable by conventional MRI. For example, the protein content of tissue can be imaged using the field dependent T_1 relaxation times [UMH⁺06].

As the focus field of an MPI system can point in any direction, a pre-polarized MPI/MRI combination has the ability to direct B_0 arbitrarily. This allows an efficient utilization of the recording coils. Moreover it could solve the problem of current mapping using MRI for electrical impedance measurements in anisotropic tissue [WS08]. In conventional MRI, only one field component can be measured in the case of low frequency current density imaging [JSH89]. There a phase shift is generated by applying a current through the patient at low frequencies. This is only sensitive to the field component in the B_0-direction. Therefore it is impossible to reconstruct the full current densities. With high frequency current density imaging [SJAH95], two field components can be detected. In this technique, fields due to the currents act as MRI RF fields. Usually, eddy currents in the patient due to the B_1 field are utilized. Still, a full reconstruction of the current density is impossible.

With the proposed pre-polarized MPI/MRI combination, all field components can be measured. This allows for reconstructing the anisotropy of the tissue conductivity. Moreover, the ability to freely choose the Larmor frequency allows for using current injection frequencies, where only a minimal effect on the patient is expected but still strong tissue specific contrast is anticipated, i.e., at around 100 kHz.

As such an MPI/MRI system has the ability to rapidly change the field strength and as it is equipped with a very broad-banded receiving system, it may also be well suited for multi-nuclei MRI. As nuclei other than protons produce only relatively weak signals, the presumably low

B_0 field strength of an MPI/MRI system is not ideal. On the other hand, there are hyperpolarized techniques in MRI using xenon (^{129}Xe) [PMH$^+$08] and helium (^{3}He) [LMB$^+$99] for lung imaging and carbon (^{13}C) [GZL$^+$06] for metabolic imaging. In a hyperpolarization procedure, a tracer material with a high nuclear polarization is produced with a separate apparatus outside the scanner. The hyperpolarized material is brought to the patient and detected using a suitable MRI sequence. So the signal to noise ratio becomes independent of the field strength.

Finally, proton lung images with improved quality could be expected, as the susceptibility artifacts are much less severe at low read-out field strength.

8.2 Vascular applications

Vascular applications are attractive for MPI because available iron oxide particles like Resovist[1] are injected into the blood stream and remain there for several minutes before being absorbed by the reticuloendothelial system. If injected as a bolus, the local concentration can be quite high.

As an example, if 7 ml of a 0.5 mol/l iron oxide solution is injected as a bolus one could expect that the tracer material dilutes to about 250 ml of blood. The concentration in the blood would be 14 mmol/l.

The expected image speed and quality obtainable at such a concentration depends on the performance of the tracer material. There are mainly two cases that have to be discussed. First, an ideal tracer is used. In the second case the expected image quality of a currently available tracer material, like Resovist, has to be predicted.

In Section 6.2 a detection limit of 13 nmol(Fe)/l for a ten minute acquisition time and one millimeter voxel size has been derived. For a voxel rate of 10^6 per second, a 14 mmol/l concentration would still be 40 times the detectable concentration. Therefore, fast angiography seems to be well feasible using an ideal tracer material.

A further topic in vascular applications is the evaluation of the tissue perfusion. This means, the dynamics of the filling of small vessels in the tissues is studied. The blood volume fraction in different tissues is

---

[1]Resovist is a commercially available MRI contrast agent. The usual dose is 8 μmol/l and the maximum safe dose according to the package insert is 40 μmol/l.

typically between 2% and 10%. For an ideal tracer, this means a high (10^6) voxel rate and 1 mm resolution can be maintained.

When using Resovist as a tracer material, the signal level for a given concentration is significantly lower. In [GW05], a signal strength reflecting 3% of the theoretical value was reported. Even so, fast angiography seems to be feasible. For a perfusion measurement, either the voxel size has to be increased or the voxel rate decreased. For 2% blood volume fraction, the linear voxel size has to be increased to about 4 mm. Reducing the voxel rate to 10^5 per second would allow voxels with a linear dimension of 2.5 mm. Therefore a broad range of vascular applications should be feasible with current tracer materials as discussed in the following sections.

The sensitivity discussion above assumes simple voxel by voxel encoding. In Section 6.3 more advanced encoding mechanisms have been discussed. Therefore, even higher performance levels can be expected for many sequences and applications.

8.2.1 Cardiovascular

Several imaging modalities are currently used for the assessment of blood supply of the heart, the coronaries, and the heart function. They are:

Catheter angiography: This is the gold standard for stenosis detection and assessment. A catheter is inserted into a vessel at the extremities and guided to the aortic arch where a bolus of an X-ray contrast agent is then administered, filling the coronaries with a high concentration. 2D X-ray transmission images are taken where the stenosis can be seen directly. If a treatable stenosis is found, a dilatation can be performed immediately, although in a large part of the patient population, no treatment is performed.

CT angiography: A bolus of an X-ray contrast agent is injected intravenously and a multi-slice CT is recorded when the bolus has reached the coronaries. Due to lower resolution, the assessment of a stenosis in CT is not as reliable as in the catheter angiography, but it is less invasive. Functional parameters, such as stroke volume, may also be extracted from the CT data.

Nuclear perfusion test: A radioactive potassium analogue (i.e., a molecule mimicking the physiological properties of potassium) PET or SPECT tracer is injected. The tracer is taken up by the perfused and vital heart muscle and an image of the 3D distribution is recorded. The test is done both in the rest state and during physical or chemical stress. A lower concentration in some region during the stress test indicates a relevant stenosis, i.e., a stenosis that is not sufficiently bypassed by another vessel. The finding of relevant stenosis is a good indication that the patient would benefit from some sort of intervention.

Ultrasound test: The differences in heart wall motion during rest and (chemically induced) stress are recorded. A lower perfusion may result in a reduced local motion of the myocardium during the stress condition. The finding of a motion anomaly justifies more invasive diagnostic measures eventually leading to a decision for therapy.

In addition to the methods described above, some more tests and imaging methods exist that address other aspects of heart disease, such as the imaging of scar tissue after an infarction.

Judging from the estimates in the beginning of this vascular section, it seems possible for MPI to play a role in the imaging of heart diseases, as it can combine the information of many of the methods above in one examination without the need for ionizing radiation. A cardiac imaging procedure with an MPI/MRI combination could be implemented as follows:

The patient is placed in the scanner and the position of the heart and large vessels is verified using a low-resolution MRI scan. Using a low dosage bolus, the precise position of the heart chambers, the large vessels and a first, low resolution image of the large coronary arteries are acquired. Using a second, more highly concentrated bolus, precise values of the inner wall movement, the stroke volume, and maybe the heart valve function are recorded. When the bolus reaches the coronaries, the scanner is switched to a special sequence where the previously acquired information of the coronaries is used to scan only that part of the heart with high spatial and temporal resolution. As the scanner may be able to follow single fluctuations of the tracer material, not only may the morphology be extracted from the data, but also the flow speed and the relative intensity of the signal along the coronary arteries. Using this information, it may be possible to precisely assess the degree of the stenosis. After the passage through the coronaries, the inflow, the maximum concentration, and the outflow characteristics of the tracer in the myocardium may be recorded. As the magnetic particles are not absorbed until after a few minutes, mainly by the liver, the imaging procedure may be repeated while chemically induced or physical stress is applied.

The final goal would be to develop an MPI scanner to the state where also catheter procedures can be performed. This would reduce the X-ray exposure of the patient and the medical staff. To reach this goal, catheters must be equipped with markers to track them by MPI. Also stents and other devices need MPI visible coatings to track their position and assess their proper function (e.g., to assess the full expansion of a stent).

8.2.2 Neurovascular

The most important neurovascular disease is stroke. To find a role for MPI in stroke care is difficult, as it is already addressed adequately by CT and MRI. Furthermore, MPI can not assist in all the decisions that have to be taken. The only curative treatment in a stroke scenario is a treatment with thrombolytic drugs. As these drugs have potentially severe or even fatal side-effect, it is necessary to assess whether the patient will suffer from such side effects and whether the patient will benefit from the treatment. So the first step is to decide, if the patient encountered an ischemic stroke, where a blood clot can be dissolved, or if a hemorrhagic stroke, where a bleeding leads to a reduced blood supply or a brain swelling and a thrombolysis would not be beneficial and, indeed, would often be fatal.

With MPI it is probably not possible to decide between these two types of stroke. While an active bleeding could be seen with MPI, it is probably impossible to see a bleeding that has already stopped. But this can be seen both with CT and MRI.

If a ischemic stroke is diagnosed, the next question to answer is, if there is some affected brain tissue that is not dead, but ill perfused (penumbra). An increase in the blood flow could save this penumbra. In MRI, this question is answered with a relatively good degree of certainty, by comparison of a perfusion and a diffusion image [MB07].

In CT the penumbra is identified using the quantitative perfusion of a X-ray contrast agent [MB07].

So, MPI can only play a role in stroke care, if it is combined with a sufficient good MRI to exclude hemorrhagic stroke. Then, MPI could give the same type of information as CT. Together with the MRI images, this may lead to a more accurate and potentially faster stroke assessment.

Additionally, stroke therapy monitoring scenario is discussed in the red blood cell labelling section (Section 8.6.1).

8.3 Gastrointestinal

Some fraction of the gastrointestinal tract can be inspected using endoscopes. No tomographic imaging method can beat the quality of these images. With cameras to be swallowed, it is now even possible to image the small intestine. Nevertheless, there may still be reasons for tomographic imaging.

Applications may be seen in the imaging of the colon, where endoscopy is unpleasant for the patient and the gut lavage is time consuming. Other applications may be in the field of suspected or possible (incomplete) bowel obstruction, a video-capsule imaging may be contraindicated. Therefore native and contrast enhanced X-ray and CT are involved in the diagnosis of small bowel diseases like Crohn's disease or ileus and bowel obstruction. Here, the use of MPI could reduce the radiation dosage. The absence of radiation would enable image acquisition for longer times, which would allow for a better assessment of the peristalsis and therefore maybe a better diagnosis.

It can also be speculated that the possibility of a continuous acquisition of high-resolution images could facilitate a virtual colonoscopy without the need for inflating the colon. If the stool is orally stained with iron oxide and a diet is used which avoids millimeter sized solid components, it may be possible to image all parts of the colon successively in a dilated state. This may allow for the detection of polyps as one example.

8.4 Lung

In the field of lung imaging, MPI may contribute to the ventilation, the perfusion imaging and the angiography of the lung. Lung perfusion is currently done using contrast enhanced CT or with SPECT. The replacement of the CT perfusion with MPI is straight forward, as the MPI tracer and the CT contrast agent have the same inflow/outflow kinetics. In SPECT lung perfusion, $10\,\mu$m to $150\,\mu$m radioactively labelled particles are intravenously injected and get stuck in the perfused area of the lung. This enrichment mechanism of the tracer may have some advantage in certain applications [PSCLM07] and may also be mimicked by MPI. The maximum number of particles is about 700000. Assuming a particle size of $70\,\mu$m, an iron concentration in the particles of $1\,$mol/l and a total lung volume of $5\,$l, the average iron concentration in the lung would be $25\,\mu$mol/l. This should be easily measurable at a resolution of 2 to $3\,$mm. A higher resolution is not useful, as the statistical variations of the number of particles in a voxel would become too high. At this concentration, MPI would be able to image the lung in a few minutes, which is substantially faster than the SPECT measurement.

The other topic in lung imaging is the assessment of the ventilation. Together with perfusion, it plays a key role in the diagnosis of lung embolism. Ventilation studies can be performed with CT [WHS+77] [HC05], hyperpolarized noble gas MRI [MRCBC08] or with SPECT/scintigraphy [PSCLM07], which is the most common method. There, either a radioactive gas ([81m]Kr or ^{133}Xe) or an aerosol containing ^{99m}Tc is inhaled. Again, the later may be mimicked by MPI. To reach an average concentration of $100\,\mu$mol/l in a 5 liter lung, one would need to inhale $1\,$ml of Resovist as an aerosol. Again, this would allow a scan time of a few seconds in comparison to several minutes in SPECT.

8.5 RES imaging/direct inflammation imaging

Imaging the activity of the reticulo-endothelial system (RES) was the original goal of Resovist. The only application realized with MRI was the imaging of liver lesions, i.e., regions in the liver where no uptake takes place. Directly imaging other parts of high uptake-activity could become an option with the increased sensitivity of MPI. However, liver uptake is fast and it is not clear now if a significant uptake can be detected elsewhere. Applications may lie in the detection of inflammation if the detection is feasible at all.

8.6 Cell labelling

Cell labelling is a very broad field with only a few clinical applications today but high hopes for future applications. Many different types of cells can be labelled. Here, only three examples should be given.

8.6.1 Red blood cell labelling

Red blood cells (RBCs) are by far the largest fraction of the solid components in human blood. In fact, blood is composed of almost 50 % red blood cells. RBCs can be labelled with radioactive tracers for SPECT imaging. These labelled cells can be used as a "blood pool agent" with long circulation time, i.e., a tracer that highlights solely the blood vessels. Applications are in the area of the determination of the local blood volume, e.g., in hemangiomas [ZYS+05]. A further application is the detection of bleedings in the intestine [ZOS+08] [How06].

There are techniques that allow for the labelling of red blood cells with iron oxide [ASM+08]. Due to the high abundance of the RBCs, it does not seem to be difficult to reach a high local concentration in the blood exceeding 1 mmol/l. So, fast imaging seems to be possible as discussed in Section 8.2. An interesting application might be the functional imaging of the brain, where local changes in blood volume are related to regional activity. Due to the long lifetime of the RBCs (up to three months), a constant labelling grade over the measuring time can be assumed. But the long lifetime of the RBCs may militate against this application, as the iron oxide in the blood would interfere for a long time with MRI and other MPI examinations. So either a method to control the RBC lifetime has to be developed or applications with lower local concentrations should be addressed.

Such an application could be the monitoring of the progress of chemotherapy by repeatedly measuring a tumor's blood volume. For this, a 100 μmol/l concentration in the blood pool should facilitate a measurement of 1 liter tumor volume in less than a minute assuming

$(5\,\text{mm})^3$ voxels. This assumes labelling with Resovist, an average of 2% blood in the tumor, and a simple voxel by voxel encoding.

A further application of red blood cell labelling would be the monitoring of stroke patients. After a stroke, the probability of bleeding is high either because the stroke is already a hemorrhagic stroke or because it has occured during the normal progression (or therapy—thrombolysis) of an ischemic stroke. A bleeding requires immediate action and hence monitoring would be beneficial. MPI could detect small amounts of labelled blood leaking out of the vasculature. As the spacial resolution required for this application is only about 1 cm, the scanner could be a quite simple device, making permanent imaging economically feasible.

8.6.2 White blood cell labelling

White blood cell labelling is currently used together with SPECT imaging [WMB+95]. During this procedure, white blood cells are separated and a sub fraction, the granulocytes, are selectively labelled with a ^{99m}Tc compound. After re-injection, these cells migrate into the inflammations and are imaged there.

To determine if MPI could play a role in the imaging of white blood cells, some assumptions have to be made. The assumptions are based on a scenario to use the white cell labelling to assess Crohn's disease. It is assumed that there are 4000 granulocytes in each μl of blood, 100 ml of blood is collected, and each cell is labelled with 5 pg of iron. The performance of Resovist is assumed for the contrast agent. After re-injection of the cells, it is assumed that the material is equally distributed over 5 liters of tissue, inspired by the images in [WMB+95] showing the distribution of white blood cells in th small intestine using SPECT. As a result, the local concentration is 7 μmol/l. According to the estimate in Section 8.2, a whole-body scan with such a concentration should be performed in a minute at a voxel size of $(5\,\text{mm})^3$.

When imaging the gut, almost the total patient volume has to be scanned. There may be other applications where the ability of MPI to scan a sub-volume is beneficial in terms of reducing scan time or increase image resolution.

8.6.3 Stem cell labelling

Stem cell labelling is the most challenging topc in the cell imaging, as it is necessary to localize only a few cells. In principle, a single cell should be visible with MPI, as the detection limit was estimated to 1 pg (see Section 6.2) and cells can be labelled with up to 10 pg of iron. However, some technical challenges remain. For an averaging over an extended time, the background signal of the scanner must be low and extremely constant. The background signal is generated by unwanted non-linearities in the scanner hardware. The amplitudes and phases of such harmonics usually drift, making a subtraction difficult. In addition, the currently available tracer material performs at best with 3 % of the theoretical signal intensity therefore an optimized tracer would be needed. Currently there are no widespread clinical applications of stem cell labelling and imaging.

8.7 Sentinel lymph node imaging

The sentinel lymph nodes are the lymph nodes near a tumor to which the interstitial fluid of the tumor is drained. If a tumor forms metastases it is likely that they occur in the sentinel lymph nodes first. So if a tumor is resected, it is an option to only resect the sentinel lymph nodes and examine them histologically instead of resecting all lymph nodes in the vicinity. If no tumor cells are found in the lymph nodes, no further action needs to be taken. In the other case, all nearby lymph nodes have to be resected as in traditional surgery. The advantage of the sentinel lymph node procedure is a potentially higher quality of life for the patient. The procedure is most common in the treatment of mamma carcinoma.

To find the sentinel lymph nodes, typically a tracer containing a blue dye and a radioactive colloid is injected into and in the rim of a mama carcinoma. The distribution of the fluid is imaged by a gamma camera before surgery to identify the sentinel lymph nodes. During surgery a Geiger counter and the blue dye are used to find the marked lymph nodes.

It is likely that a whole body MPI scanner could image the distribution of intratumoral injected iron oxide colloid, like the gamma camera in the current procedure. But it would be more appealing to have a small hand-held device to do the imaging. Luckily, the field geometries needed for MPI allow for a field generator applied from only one side of the object [GW04b] [SKB+09]. So it may be possible to construct a small hand held device that can be used instead of the current sentinel lymph node procedure.

Such devices, suitable for use during surgery, may be suitable for other applications as well. It may even be possible to mount a small MPI scanner on a (ceramic blade) scalpel and generate an acoustic feedback when the blade is near a vessel, provided the vessel contains blood that is labelled with magnetic nano-particles.

8.8 Hyperthermia

Hyperthermia using a magnetic fluid is an experimental therapy for cancer [JSW+97]. A magnetic fluid is directly injected into the tumor. Then, an external magnetic field is applied and the magnetic fluid heats up. As the magnetic material stays near the tumor, the heating is localized, minimizing the damage to surrounding tissue.

In hyperthermia, MPI may provide an additional benefit by localizing the heat generation. If a selection field is provided, the heat generation will be restricted to the area that is covered by the field free point movement. This may be useful in cases when the magnetic fluid leaks out of the tumor. A selection field could also be used to heat the tumor more homogeneously, if the magnetic particles are heterogeneously distributed. In addition MPI may monitor the distribution of the magnetic particles and the power dissipation. With methods described in Section 9.4, it may even be possible to monitor the temperature.

Theoretically, MPI would allow for localized hyperthermia even if the tracer is distributed homogeneously in the body. But this might not be feasible because of the high dosages needed. For mild hyperthermia, local power absorption of $50\,\mathrm{W/l}$ seems to be necessary [WGJ+06]. The maximum heat can be generated if the magnetization curve forms a rectangular hysteresis (see Fig. 4.4 middle row, left), having a half width equal to the applied field. So,

$$P_{\mathrm{max}} = 4\mu_0 f m H.$$

Here, f is the frequency, H the external magnetic field and m the saturation magnetic dipole moment. 1 mol of iron in magnetite has a dipole moment of $7\,\text{Am}^2$. At a well tolerable $7\,\text{mT}\mu_0^{-1}$ external field amplitude and at a frequency of $100\,\text{kHz}$, the maximum possible power is $20\,\text{kW/mol}$. So, the local concentration for $50\,\text{W/l}$ needs to be $2.5\,\text{mmol/l}$. This is about half a liter of a $0.5\,\text{molar}$ iron oxide suspension like Resovist in a $70\,\text{kg}$ patient. The $2.5\,\text{molar}$ concentration is still well below the LD50 for rats [LBF+97], but the material is not close to the theoretical heating efficiency. The values reported in [WGJ+06] lead to about $340\,\text{W/mol}$ of heat generation at the field and frequency values used above. So a magnetic fluid hyperthermia using a systemic injection is only possible if the properties of the magnetic material are vastly improved.

9 Potential further developments and applications

For the applications listed in Chapter 8, it is very likely that an MPI scanner can provide useful images with existing contrast agents. The unknown part is if the images are good enough and the procedure is fast and cheap enough to compete with the existing modalities. Now, potential applications will be discussed that need contrast agents that are not yet available, or that use physical principles that exist, but where the practical feasibility in biological tissue is not known.

9.1 Tissue intrinsic contrast MPI

The assumption that human tissue does not contain ferromagnetic material does not seem to be true for all circumstances. There is some evidence that biogenic iron oxide is linked to Alzheimer's disease [HPKD03] or tumors [BHW+06] [KYK97]. The reported magnetization levels of the order of $1\,\mathrm{mAm^2/kg}$ lie well above the detection limit of MPI. From the current perspective it is unclear if the particles are efficient for MPI applications. They could be too small or too anisotropic to generate a useful signal. It is also not clear if the finding of MPI-active biogenic nano-particles would have any significance for diagnosis, i.e., if it would change the therapy or shift the diagnosis to an earlier stage of the disease.

9.2 Targeted imaging

Targeted imaging is the most obvious application that can not be addressed with the contrast agents available today. The basic idea is to attach a molecule to the magnetic particles that binds specifically to tissue. Antibodies may serve as such specific binding molecules.

The detection of radioactively labelled antibodies is called "radioimmunoscintigraphic" and is currently used in some SPECT oncology procedures [JSR+93].

Here, MPI can not be used in the same way as the nuclear methods. The reason lies in the size of the magnetic particle. The hydrodynamic diameter of a suitable MPI tracer particle is on the order of 50 nm which is considerably larger than the size of immunoglobulins. So the pharmacokinetics is severely altered. In particular, it is unlikely that the particles can leave the vessel system without the help of immune cells. So, targeted imaging with MPI is basically limited to vascular targets, i.e., antigens that are displayed in the vessel system. A variety of such targets does exist [WCC+07], but there is no widespread clinical use, yet. MPI should be sensitive enough to be used in such applications, as they are currently addressed with MRI, and a fully optimized MPI would be much more sensitive to iron oxide than MRI.

9.3 Lung diffusion imaging

In lung imaging, there might be more relevant parameters than pure ventilated air space as discussed in Section 8.4. The diffusion parameters of gases may reveal deeper insight into the structure of the lung [SY08] [WCY+06] [PMH+08], revealing potentially important information for asthma, emphysema and chronic obstructive pulmonary disease [MH02]. The apparent diffusion coefficient is linked to the average distance to the lung surface, thus a large diffusion indicates enlarged lung structures, e.g., enlarged alveoli in an emphysema.

MPI may also offer a way to obtain information revealing the lung structure. Such a contrast could be based on the signal generation in air space due to fast Brownian rotation mechanisms. In Chapter 4.3, Brownian rotation was excluded as an effective mechanism for signal generation in liquid suspensions. The viscosity of air is only 18 μPas, leading to more than 50 times the magnetization speed of suspensions in water. Therefore, it should be possible to efficiently detect magnetic particles in air space even if the anisotropy is so high that the Neel process is blocked. When a particle reaches the lung's surface, the Brownian rotation is also blocked and the MPI signal vanishes.

The particles will reach the lung surface by diffusion. The speed of the diffusion may be estimated by the Einstein formula:

$$\bar{x} = \sqrt{\frac{2k_BTt}{3\pi r\eta}}$$

Here, $\bar{x}$ is the mean travel distance, r the particle radius, η the viscosity of the medium, and t the time. For air viscosity and 40 nm particle diameter, the travel distance in one second is about 50 μm. This is to be compared with the typical alveolar air space of 50 to 250 μm in healthy lung tissue. In emphysema, the air space is enlarged, which should be detectable as a change in the signal decay time. As a benefit to the patient, it is probably not necessary to hold the breath for longer than 5 seconds.

The estimates just performed assumed particles with completely blocked Neel rotation. Nevertheless, it may be possible to use the change in signal shape when particles with only slight anisotropy get attached to the lung surface. When such particles attach to the lung surface, the signal is not quenched completely, but the amplitude and phases of the harmonics change, i.e., the shape of the generated signal. Therefore, existing iron oxide nano-particles based contrast agents (e.g., Resovist) may be used for this application, provided they can be sprayed in a fine enough aerosol.

9.4 Temperature imaging

It might be possible to use the anisotropy of the particles to image the temperature or other physical or chemical parameters [Gle04a]. The basic idea behind this is that a shell around a magnetic particle melts at a specific temperature. In the molten state, the particle shows a faster Brownian rotation than in the solid state. These differences might be measured using a suitable MPI sequence. A simple sequence might be:

- Excite a voxel with a small FFP movement in one direction for a sufficiently long time.

The particles will align with their easy axis in the direction of the drive field and the signal will be large.

- Switch the drive field to the orthogonal direction.

The signal will be initially lower, as the easy axis of the particles is now perpendicular to the drive field. But the particles will re-orient to the new drive field direction and the signal will increase to the original level. The rise time of the signal is a measure of the temperature.

For other parameters, like pH or oxygen pressure, a coating material might be found that changes volume (swells, shrinks) when the parameter is changed. The change in size would also change the speed of the geometric rotation, leading to a different MPI signal.

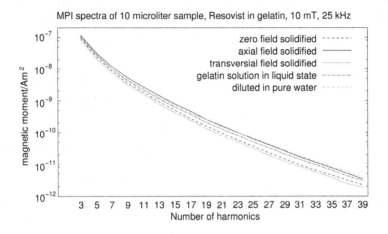

MPI spectra of 10 microliter sample, Resovist in gelatin, 10 mT, 25 kHz

Figure 9.1: MPI spectra of Resovist in gelatin solutions. The samples differ in the state of the gelatin (solid/liquid), but not in the concentration, which is about 2 %.

The effect of an inhibited rotational freedom is shown in the MPI spectra in Fig. 9.1. A MPI spectrum is the response of a small sample in the "neutral" position of the FFP, using a one-dimensional drive field. As the selection field does not have any effect on the sample (the field is zero), it is usually omitted. The spectrometer results are displayed as Fourier amplitudes of the magnetization (not as induced voltage).

It can be seen from the figure that the signal is high if the particles are aligned with the drive field direction and low if unaligned or even aligned in perpendicular direction. The difference in signal intensity at high frequencies is more than double. So the effect should be quite easily detectable, even if the magnetic particles and the sequence are not optimized for this application.

The ability to measure the absolute temperature of tissue may be useful in oncology. Tumors are reported to show an increase of about 1 K in temperature relative to the surrounding tissue [SCM+01] [SCP+03]. The temperature can also be heterogeneously distributed in the tumor tissue [GJG82]. Moreover, the efficiency of a chemotherapy may affect the temperature of the tumor early [NOB+86] and thus MPI might be used to measure the efficiency of the therapy.

9.5 MPI-acoustic imaging and Elastography

Elastography is a method to determine the elastic properties of tissue by moving the tissue with a low-frequency elastic wave and determining the tissue movement with an imaging modality [FEP+95]. The imaging modality needs sufficient resolution to allow the detection of the small movements due to the acoustic wave. MPI may serve as a suitable imaging modality in this context. The advantage over MRI would be its faster acquisition speed.

MPI may also offer a method to determine the pressure of high frequency ultrasound in the tissue using pressure sensitive tracer materials [Gle04c]. Such a tracer could be similar to currently used ultrasound contrast agents. They are essentially stabilized gas bubbles of about $10\,\mu m$ size. It may be possible to place iron oxide particles in the shell. If the sound wave squeezes the bubbles, the distance between the iron oxide particles changes leading to a different magnetization curve. Thus, the magnetization of the bubbles changes synchronously with the sound wave and as a result, a magnetic signal can be measured. The effect occurs only near the FFP, as otherwise all the magnetic particles are already saturated and a change in particle–particle interaction does not induce a change in magnetization.

The measurement of the ultrasound pressure field could be interesting, as it allows for the extraction of more elastic parameters than ultrasound alone. Most interestingly, the absolute sound velocity becomes accessible leading to a potentially interesting soft-tissue contrast.

An alternative way to determine the sound speed in the tissue would be to generate a sound wave using MPI. This is also possible and does not even need a special tracer material [GWB10]. The gradient field imposes a force on the magnetic material. The direction of the force points away from the FFP. If the FFP moves over the object, regions with sudden change in stress are generated that emit a sound wave. The sound wave can be detected at the surface of the patient. In the above publication, the detection limit was estimated to about $4\,\mu$mol/l for a 1 second acquisition.

An alternative way to generate sound from the particles is the thermo-acoustic effect. If the particles re-magnetize, heat is dissipated. This results in a slight temperature increase of the surrounding tissue, which expands. The rapid expansion leads to the emission of a pressure wave. Assuming ideal particles that change magnetization stepwise at a field of $2\,\mathrm{mT}\mu_0^{-1}$ at an iron concentration of $100\,\mu$mol/l, the expected pressure temperature increase is $7 \cdot 10^{-10}\,$K. Using the thermal expansion coefficient of water at $20°$ C of $2.1 \cdot 10^{-4}\,\mathrm{K}^{-1}$ and its compression modulus of $2\,$GPa, the expected pressure pulse has an intensity of $300\,\mu$Pa. In comparison, the thermal noise in water for a 1 mm^2 detector is $160\,\mu$Pa$/\sqrt{\mathrm{Hz}}$ (derived from [FH01]). So the thermo-acoustic detection of magnetic nano-particles is much less sensitive than the gradient method but has the advantage that the signal is influenced by thermal and mechanical properties of the tissue in the direct neighborhood of the particles. Furthermore, the sensitivity could be increased using particles with a very high coercivity.

Yet another method to couple MPI with ultrasound is to utilize an orientation-dependent ultrasound scattering of nano-particles or nano-particle labelled red blood cells. This is similar to the electrophysiology imaging described later (see Section 9.8).

9.6 Pulmonary artery pressure

The pressure in the pulmonary arteries is not directly accessible from the outside. Therefore, a catheter procedure is the most reliable way to measure it [FFC$^+$09]. However, MPI might offer a much less invasive method for its determination.

In the previous section, a pressure sensitive tracer was mentioned, but it is not suitable for measuring blood pressure: The blood pressure change in the pulmonary arteries is on the order of $10\,$hPa, while typical diagnostic ultrasound pressures are on the order of $1\,$MPa. To increase the sensitivity, the pressure measuring device must possess a low stiffness in order to show a strong size and shape change at the given pressure change. The stiffness of the gas filled bubble is given by the gas pressure. To change the volume by a factor of 2, it is necessary to apply a pressure equivalent to the pressure in the gas bubble. To construct a much softer device, it could be useful to build a miniature evacuated vessel similar to the aneroid cell in a barometer. The cell can consist of ferromagnetic material and the change in anisotropy can be measured. It might also be possible to measure the pressure dependent change in the resonance frequency of the device.

As it is likely that the device has to be calibrated individually, the device must be large enough to be imaged individually. So, it should be as large as possible. Particles with $100\,\mu$m diameter seem to be small enough that no relevant lung embolisms are expected [PSCLM07]. If such a device contains $1\,\%$ iron, the mass of the iron is about $40\,$ng. With such an amount of iron, the anisotropy should be accessible in a few milliseconds. If the device is made of bio-degradable polymers and pure iron, it could be fully metabolized within days or weeks [PHS$^+$06].

There is already evidence that a pressure sensing device could work. In Fig. 9.2, the MPI spectra of Mu-metal foils are displayed. The foils of size $2\,$mm$\times1\,$mm$\times2.7\,\mu$m are aligned with the long axis parallel to the drive field. The spikes labelled with "together" and "reunited" refer to a situation where the foils are close together, i.e., forming a $2\,$mm$\times1\,$mm$\times5.4\,\mu$m structure. In the "separated" case, the foils have a separation of $\approx1\,$mm. In this case, the spectral intensities of the higher harmonics are higher almost by a factor of 10 . This is to be expected, as the effective demagnetization factor is lower than in the compact ("together") structure, which means a steeper magnetization curve. By exploiting this effect, it is likely that an MPI based pressure measuring device can be constructed if the separation of two magnetic foils is controlled by the external pressure.

It should also be noted that the MPI signal efficiency of the Mu-metal foils is quite high. The saturation magnetization of this nickel-iron alloy is about $0.8\,$Tμ_0^{-1}, which means a total magnetic dipole moment of the two foils of $7\,\mu$Am^2. Assuming a perfect square wave describing the magnetization, an amplitude of $2.3\,\mu$Am^2 is expected in the third harmonics. The observed value in Fig. 9.2 is not much less, indicating the feasibility of the millisecond read-out time.

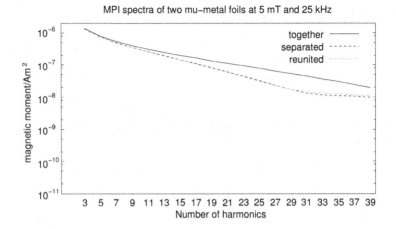

Figure 9.2: MPI spectra of two Mu-metal foils $(2\,\text{mm}\times1\,\text{mm}\times2.7\,\mu\text{m})$ close together or separated by $1\,\text{mm}$. In the first measurement, labelled "together", the foils are close to each other. The data labelled with "separated" reflect the state where the foils are separated by one millimeter. The last data, labelled "reunited" represent a control measurement, where the foils are put in close contact again.

9.7 Object tracking and manipulation

The hardware of a fully electromagnetic MPI scanner, i.e., in which all fields are generated by electromagnets, would be able to produce gradient fields and also homogeneous fields with arbitrary directions. This was discussed for the combination with MRI in Section 8.1. This capability can be used to steer a catheter in a similar way as is done with a Stereotaxis system [EOL+04]. In such a system, the catheter or guidewire is equipped with magnetic material (soft magnetic or permanent magnetic) at the distal end. A homogeneous field orients the magnetic material and can be used to rotate the tip in any direction. With this capability, it is possible to guide the catheter through the vessel tree or press it against the heart wall as needed for electrophysiology mapping or ablation. Due to the lack of an X-ray system which would allow for a compactness of the magnet assembly, the field strength and switching speed of an MPI system would be much higher than that of the current Stereotaxis system.

An MPI system can also act as an imaging device and a catheter tracking system. For the tracking part, small soft magnetic objects along the catheter are sufficient. While imaging and tracking, the force on the Stereotaxis catheter alters, so only selected periods of imaging, interleaved with manipulation, are possible and probably sufficient, given the speed of MPI.

The strong field gradients of an MPI system could also be used to drag a small magnetic object through the vessel tree. Using Stokes law, the speed of a magnetic sphere of radius r in a magnetic gradient G is given by

$$v = \frac{2}{9} \frac{\mu_0 M G r^2}{\eta}.$$

Here, M is the average magnetization of the sphere and η the viscosity of the medium. A sphere with $200\,\mu$m might be small enough to be only a little hazard when blocking a small blood vessels. For a useful device, similar to the one described for pressure measurement, the magnetization can reach 10% of magnetite magnetization. An MPI system could exhibit a gradient of $3\,\mathrm{T}\mu_0^{-1}/\mathrm{m}$. Blood has a complex viscosity behavior. $6\,\mathrm{mPas}$ may be taken as an average viscosity, motivated from [MZX+05]. With these numbers, the speed of the device would exceed $20\,\mathrm{cm/s}$. Assuming a cardiac output of $5\,\mathrm{l/min}$ and an aorta diameter of $2.5\,\mathrm{cm}$, the blood flow speed would be $17\,\mathrm{cm/s}$. Consequently, it would be possible to drag such a device against the fastest blood flow in the body. So, it might also be possible to move the pressure measuring device to record data at different positions for an extended period of time. This might allow evaluating the pressure drop along a stenosis.

Steering a small device to a specific location can be useful in therapy, too. A "device" containing a lysis drug could be steered directly to the stenosis, maximizing the effect while minimizing side effects. The device could be a solid or liquid mixture of the drug and iron oxide nano-particles in a slowly dissolving shell. The steering ability could also be used to place magnetic brachytherapy seeds in a tumor through the vessel system.

9.8 Electrophysiology imaging

MPI relies on having a field free point and a material exhibiting a non-linearity near zero field. The original idea was to use the nonlinearity of the magnetization curve of magnetic material near a zero magnetic field. But there are other nonlinearities that can be used. One that has already been discussed is the non-linearity of the force on magnetic particles as explained in Section 9.5.

In another example, the effect of the magnetic field on the resistivity will be exploited. There are several physical effects where a magnetic field influences the resistivity of a material. The magneto-resistive effect in ferromagnetic materials generated by the spin-dependent scattering of electrons (magneto-resistance, anisotropic magneto-resistance, giant magneto-resistance, ...) gained widespread applications, e.g., in hard drives for information storage. Exploiting these effects in a biological context does not seem to be promising, because the resistivity change of the pure ferromagnetic material is only a few per cent and the resistivity of the ferromagnetic material is very low compared to tissue resistivity. In addition, the volume fraction of the magnetic material is very low in medical applications. So the tissues resistivity change is expected to be too small for medical applications.

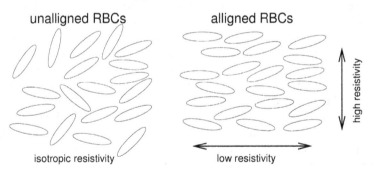

Figure 9.3: Aligned red blood cells (RBCs) produce an anisotropic con-
          ductivity of the blood. In the aligned case, the current in
          the direction of the cells short axis has to travel a longer dis-
          tance in the plasma than the current in long axis direction.

It seems more promising to exploit the orientation of red blood cells

(RBCs). RBCs are disk shaped with an aspect ratio of about 4. Non-oriented blood cells will show an isotropic resistance, while oriented blood cells will show a large anisotropy in the conductivity (see Fig. 9.3). The lipid membrane of the cells can be viewed as an insulation for low frequencies. As the volume fraction of RBCs is almost 50%, the orientation effect is expected to be several 10%.

The manipulation of the orientation can be achieved by labelling the red blood cells with iron oxide as described earlier (see Section 8.6.1). Due to the demagnetization factor, the cells prefer to have their long axis aligned in the field direction. The orientation of the magnetic field changes rapidly near the field free point. Therefore, it is possible to change the anisotropy of the conductivity locally.

Such an effect can be used in several ways. It may be used to measure the impedance of tissue. For this, an external voltage source is applied to the patient. The change of the current during the movement of the FFP is recorded. Using a suitable reconstruction algorithm, the tissues impedance values may be derived from the measured signals.

Another use can be the measurement of the local electrical activity of tissue, especially of heart tissue. Here, the electrical activity is measured at the skin of the patient and the change of the activity is correlated with the movement of the field free point.

To illustrate such electrophysiology imaging, it can be assumed that there is one electric dipole (nearby plus and minus pole) in the patient. This dipole generates a voltage at the surface of the patient which can be measured. In addition, it is assumed that the electrical conductivity is increased at the position of the field free point. If the field free point is far away from the electric dipole, the voltage at the surface of the patient is virtually unchanged. When the field free point reaches the dipole, the electric field is short-circuited and the voltage drops. All electric activities can be decomposed into electric dipoles. Thus, it is possible to move the field free point, and hence the high conductivity region, over the whole volume of interest and thereby map the electric activity.

Weather these applications are feasible depends on the degree of orientation that can be reached. The main counteracting effect is the rotation of the RBCs by the shear forces in the vessels.

Instead of using a contrast agent, it may also be possible to use a device which is moved and tracked by MPI. The movement of such a device was described earlier in Section 9.7. For ECG mapping, the device could simply be a tiny conductive and ferromagnetic wire with a length of a few mm. If moved through the heart chambers, it would modulate the blood conductivity and therefore the external ECG signal. Using tiny iron rods in degradable polymers, the device could disintegrate within a few hours after the application.

9.9 Light modulation

In addition to the conductivity, the orientation of red blood cells can also alter the scattering properties of tissue as used in pulse oxymeters [SFK07]. Therefore, it should be possible to use the localized change in the optical properties of the tissue to increase the resolution of diffuse optical tomography. This may be useful for imaging the oxygen concentration in deep lying tumors. But as discussed in Section 2.4, the penetration depth of light in human tissue is limited to several centimeters, which limits the number of accessible tumors.

A second way to use the MPI encoding mechanism for optical imaging is to use a dye that is sensitive to magnetic fields. Dyes exist that change their fluorescence yield in weak magnetic fields below $5\,\mathrm{mT}\mu_0^{-1}$ [PBSA92]. The image formation process simply involves the movement of the field free point over the volume of interest and recording the fluorescence light intensity. The recorded signal reflects the product of excitation light intensity at the field free point, the fluorescence light attenuation from the FFP to the detector, and the dye concentration. Using a variety of light sources and detectors, it is possible to separate these contributions, yielding images of dye concentration and light absorption and scattering. Medical applications would need a dye that is active in tissue and has suitable enrichment properties.

MPI fluorescence yield imaging could also be used for microscopy. In contrast to magnetic nano-particles, these dyes are not significantly attracted to the magnetic poles, even if very high magnetic gradients are applied. Therefore, very strong selection field gradients can be used exceeding $10^6\,\mathrm{T}\mu_0^{-1}/\mathrm{m}$. Such strong gradients are formed between permanent magnetic poles with a separation of about $10\,\mu\mathrm{m}$. The resolution would be the ratio between the onset of the magnetic field effect (below $5\,\mathrm{mT}\mu_0^{-1}$) and the gradient of the selection field. Therefore resolutions on the order of 10 nm seem to be possible, this being significantly higher than the light's wavelength. In contrast to other methods of achieving sub wavelength resolution, such a microscopy would also work in turbid media.

9.10 X-ray modulation

Not only optical light could be modulated using the local change of the scattering cross section or angle. The geometric rotation of magnetic objects could also modulate X-ray scattering and absorption. If particles with a fixed correlation between the easy axis and the crystal lattice were available, an effect of field free point movement on the coherent scattering could be expected. Unfortunately, the scattering coefficients are small and a medical application does not seem to be likely.

No effect on the X-ray absorption is expected from nano-particles. The particles are so small that the X-ray intensity on the illuminated side and the opposite side are virtually identical. Even if the particles are needle shaped, the orientation does not change the number of absorbed photons.

The situation changes if the particles become larger, reaching the absorption length for X-rays. Then needles absorb less photons when illuminated from the tip. In tungsten, the inverse of the absorption coefficient for $70\,keV$ photons is $50\,\mu m$. If tungsten needles are combined with a permanent magnetic material, they could act like a miniature compass needle. The orientation of these needles can be imaged by X-ray.

Applications could be found in the localization of medical instruments and devices, such as catheters, during an X-ray guided intervention. While the position in two dimensions is easily assessed in the projection image, the third coordinate is not directly visible. Needles, together with an inhomogeneous external magnetic field, may solve the problem.

9.11 Targeted drug delivery

MPI might have more applications in therapy than localized hyperthermia. The principle of having an effect at zero field strength could also be used for targeted drug delivery. One idea is to have a tiny capsule

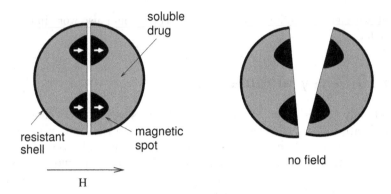

Figure 9.4: Principle of local drug delivery. Two half spheres are held
together by magnetic forces. Without an external magnetic
field, the magnetic spots loose their magnetization and the
spheres break up. The soluble drug is exposed to the blood
plasma.

consisting of half spheres (see Fig. 9.4). The half spheres are held together by soft magnetic spots consisting of many nano-particles. The
attractive force only persists as long as the spheres are in a strong magnetic field. Consequently, at the zero field spot, the halves separate and
the highly soluble drug is quickly released. To counteract leakage at
the fissure, the spheres should be as large as possible. In addition, they
must have a diameter below $10\,\mu$m to pass through all blood vessels.
For bio-compatibility, the resistant shell, protecting the curved part of
the half spheres, must also be degradable, but on a longer timescale,
to allow the capsule time to travel from the injection site to the target
region.

10 Conclusion

In the beginning of the document, the currently successful imaging techniques were analysed and a wish list of desired properties of medical tomographic imaging methods was generated. So the imaging method should:

1. provide a good resolution, i.e., type **i** or **iii** encoding mechanism (see Section 2.3).

2. be able to image at least 10 cm, probably 20 cm deep inside the tissue.

3. have the ability to use a contrast agent.

4. address a broad range of diseases.

5. not use ionizing radiation.

6. provide contrast without the use of a contrast agent.

7. permit a contrast agent with low toxicity.

8. offer high imaging speed.

9. allow a low cost examination.

In the course of this document, most of these points were addressed and could be answered positively for MPI. High resolution, penetration of the whole body and use of a contrast agent are possible. Scenarios to address several diseases have been presented. The radiation used in MPI is non-ionizing and is probably non-harmful to the patient. MPI itself is not able to acquire non contrast agent images from the patient, but it can be easily combined with magnetic resonance imaging to offer high quality anatomic and functional images.

The contrast agent used today in MPI is approved and considered safe in the dosages needed. The imaging speed is high, although it is not the highest compared to other imaging modalities. Nevertheless, due to the high flexibility in selecting the region of interest and field of view, MPI may be extremely fast in selected applications.

Predicting the cost of a new technology is not easy and was not the main focus of this document. Nevertheless it can be speculated that the procedure cost may be considerably lower than in MRI and comparable to CT. Considering the current developement state of the contrast agent, the absolute field strengths in an MPI scanner are comparable to those in an MRI machine. Therefore the intrumentation cost may be comparable. Nevertheless, the imaging procedure could be as fast as in CT, and therefore the costs of the total procedure may be much lower than for MRI, approaching those of CT.

	LF	OPT	X-ray	elast	none
LF	MPI MPI-eit MPI-eph MPI-brlx			adMPI taMPI	
OPT		eMPI MPI-lm			
X-ray			MPI-xm		
elast	MPI-p MPI-e			MPI-usm	
fluid					MPI-ht MPI-dd
none	iMPI				

Table 10.1: Magnetic particle imaging related techniques. The table is analogous to Table 2.4. The abbreviations are listed in Table 10.2.

One of the weak sides of MPI is the tracer performance. All imaging experiments performed so far used tracers with only 1% of the theoretical possible performance. Some clinical applications may be possible with this level of performance, but for a widespread acceptance of MPI, a tracer with at least ten times the current performance must be found.

In this document, numerous potential applications of an MPI scanner have been addressed. Some of them simply reproduce current imaging

MPI: Magnetic Particle Imaging The magnetic particle imaging technique as described in [GW05].

MPI-eit: MPI for Electrical Impedance tomography The magnetic particles modulate conductivity to allow for high resolution reconstruction of the electrical conductivity.

MPI-eph: MPI Electro-Physiology mapping Like MPI-eit, but physiological currents in the heart are modulated.

MPI-brlx: MPI Brownian ReLaXation measurements Measuring the particle rotation speed, e.g., for temperature imaging.

MPI-p: MPI pressure measurement Using the pressure dependent demagnetization factor to measure blood pressure in the pulmonary arteries and other vessels.

MPI-e: MPI Elastography Imaging of tissue Determination of elastic properties by measuring low-frequency displacements using MPI.

iMPI: Intrinsic MPI Imaging of iron oxide naturally occurring in tissue.

eMPI: Exciplex MPI Using magnetic field modulated fluorescence yields for optical tomography, e.g., in microscopy applications.

MPI-lm: MPI Light Modulation Using light scattering modulation near the field free point to facilitate high resolution reconstruction in diffuse optical tomography.

adMPI: Acoustically Detected MPI Detection of ultrasound emissions near the FFP trajectory.

taMPI: Thermo-Acoustic MPI Detection of thermo-acoustic emissions near the FFP trajectory.

MPI-usm: MPI UltraSound Modulation Measurement of ultrasound scattering changes near the FFP, e.g., to determine absolute sound velocities.

MPI-ht: MPI HyperThermia Confined magnetic fluid hyperthermia using a field free point.

MPI-dd: MPI Drug Delivery Deliver drugs to a specific location using effects near a field free point.

Table 10.2: Abbreviations used in Table 10.1.

methods, like the MRI mode of an MPI scanner. Some are possible
with current technology, but could be substantially improved by MPI,
such as simultaneous coronary artery and myocardium perfusion without ionizing radiation. And some are impossible as yet without surgical
intervention, such as pulmonary artery pressure determination or elec-
trophysiological imaging.

Given the broad range of possible applications of MPI, it is not easy
to decide which would be the best to start with. There are several
strategies conceivable. One of these strategies is to address a common
disease first, where imaging plays a significant role today, such as the
coronary heart diseases where X-ray based methods are dominant. If
it was shown that MPI could provide the same information as CT or
angiography, the clinical relevance would be immediately clear. On the
other hand, such a scenario leads inevitably to a turf battle which is
hard to win. The opposite scenario, i.e., addressing a disease where
imaging is not yet possible, may be a valid option for MPI, too. For
example, no imaging technology exists totay capable of acquiring high
resolution images of the heart's electric activity. MPI may do the trick
one time. Focusing on such an application has two drawbacks. First,
the research effort for realizing such applications is high and, second, it
is not evident if the gathered information justifies the imaging cost. In
my view, both approaches are needed to lead MPI to success. The first
one gives the public or private investors confidence that invested money
will pay-off and the second one may lead to a high enough incentive for
clinicians to actually start using the new and unknown scanner.

MPI should not be seen as an isolated technique. The combination
of a field free point (or line), and a material that changes properties
between zero and a low field amplitude gives rise to a considerable number of related techniques. Materials can change, e.g., their mechanicl,
electrical or optical properties in weak magnetic fields. In Table 10.1, a
list of possible imaging and therapy methods is presented which use the
various interactions. Few of them have been explored experimentally,
yet. Even with this undoubtedly incomplete list, it is immediately clear
that the invention of MPI opened a new and broad field of research.
My hope is that many researchers will bring MPI and new, related,
ideas to the stage of fruitful experiments, scanners, and applications.

In the few years since the invention of MPI, it has already been
developed to a state where in-vivo images of small animals are possible
using a physiologically tolerable contrast agent dosage. Nevertheless,

MPI has to be considered to be still in a very early state, needing several more years of development until the first images of humans can be expected.

Bibliography

[Ang58]   H. Anger. Scintillation camera. *Rev. Sci. Instrum.*, 29:27–33, 1958.

[ASM⁺08]   A. Antonelli, C. Sfara, L. Mosca, E. Manuali, and M. Magnani. New biomimetic constructs for improved in vivo circulation of superparamagnetic nanoparticles. *J Nanosci Nanotechnol*, 8(5):2270–2278, 2008.

[BHW⁺06]   F. Brem, A. Hirt, M. Winklhofer, K. Frei, Y. Yonekawa, H. Wieser, and J. Dobson. Magnetic iron compounds in the human brain: a comparison of tumour and hippocampal tissue. *J R Soc Interface.*, 3(11):833–841, 2006.

[Bow82]   T. Bowen. Radiation-induced thermoacoustic imaging, 1982.

[Cal85]   H. Callen. *Thermodynamics and an Introduction to Thermostatistics*. John Wiley and Sons, New York, 1985. ISBN 0-471-86256-8.

[CB04]   J. Clarke and A. Braginsk. *The SQUID Handbook, Vol.1: Fundamentals and Technology of SQUIDs and SQUID Systems*. Wiley-VCH, 2004. ISBN 3527402292.

[CC78]   S. Chikazumi and S. Charap. *Physics of Magnetism*. Krieger Pub Co, 1978. ISBN 0882756621.

[CCL⁺05]   R. Choe, A. Corlu, K. Lee, T. Durduran, S. Konecky, M. Grosicka-Koptyra, S. Arridge, B. Czerniecki, D. Fraker, A. DeMichele, B. Chance, M. Rosen, and A. Yodh. Diffuse optical tomography of breast cancer during neoadjuvant chemotherapy: a case study with comparison to MRI. *Med Phys.*, 32(4):1128–1139, 2005.

[CHB73]   D. Chesler, B. Hoop, and G. Brownell. Transverse section imaging of myocardium with $^{13}NH_4$. *Journal of Nuclear Medicine*, 14:623, 1973.

[CSS+80]   A. Crummy, C. Strother, J. Sackett, D. Ergun, C. Shaw, R. Kruger, C. Mistretta, W. Turnipseed, R. Lieberman, P. Myerowitz, and F. Ruzicka. Computerized fluoroscopy: digital subtraction for intravenous angiocardiography and arteriography. *AJR Am J Roentgenol*, 135(6):1131–1140, 1980.

[Dam72]   Raymond Damadian. "apparatus and method for detecting cancer in tissue", 1972.

[Dus42]   K.T. Dussik. Über die Möglichkeit hochfrequente mechanische Schwingungen als diagnostische Hilfsmittel zu verwenden. *Z. F. d. ges. Neurol. u. Psychiat.*, 174(143), 1942.

[EIJKT90] R. Edwards, M. Ibison, J. Jessel-Kenyon, and R. Taylor. Measurements of human bioluminescence. *Acupunct Electrother*, 15(2):85–94, 1990.

[EOL+04]   S. Ernst, F. Ouyang, C. Linder, K. Hertting, F. Stahl, J. Chun, H. Hachiya, D. Bänsch, M. Antz, and K. Kuck. Initial experience with remote catheter ablation using a novel magnetic navigation system: magnetic remote catheter ablation. *Circulation*, 109(12):1472–1475, 2004.

[FEP+95]   J. Fowlkes, S. Emelianov, J. Pipe, A. Skovoroda, P. Carson, R. Adler, and A. Sarvazyan. Magnetic-resonance imaging techniques for detection of elasticity variation. *Med Phys*, 22(11 Pt 1):1771–1778, 1995.

[FFC+09]   M. Fisher, P. Forfia, E. Chamera, T. Housten-Harris, H. Champion, R. Girgis, M. Corretti, and P. Hassoun. Accuracy of Doppler Echocardiography in the Hemodynamic Assessment of Pulmonary Hypertension. *Am J Respir Crit Care Med*, Jan 2009.

[FH01]   R. Farlow and G. Hayward. The minimum signal force detectable in air with a piezoelectric plate transducer. *Proc. R. Soc. Lond. A.*, 467:2741–2755, 2001.

[GJG82]   P. Gullino, R. Jain, and F. Grantham. Temperature gradients and local perfusion in a mammary carcinoma. *J Natl Cancer Inst.*, 68(3):519–533, 1982.

[GKD⁺08]   F. Gallagher, M. Kettunen, S. Day, D. Hu, J. Ardenkjaer-Larsen, R. Zandt, P. Jensen, M. Karlsson, K. Golman, M. Lerche, and K. Brindle. Magnetic resonance imaging of pH in vivo using hyperpolarized 13C-labelled bicarbonate. *nature*, 453(7197):940–943], 2008.

[Gle01]   B. Gleich. German Patent No. DE-10151778-A1, October 2001.

[Gle04a]   B. Gleich. World Patent No. WO-2004091396-A2, April 2004.

[Gle04b]   B. Gleich. World Patent No. WO-2004091397-A2, April 2004.

[Gle04c]   B. Gleich. World Patent No. WO-2004091408-A2, April 2004.

[GLG96]   S. Gabriel, R. Lau, and C. Gabriel. The dielectric properties of biological tissues: II. Measurements in the frequency range 10 Hz to 20 GHz. *Phys. Med. Biol.*, 41:2251–2269., 1996. web interface: http://niremf.ifac.cnr.it/tissprop/.

[Gob87]   H. Gobrecht, editor. *Elektrizität und Magnetismus.* Number 2 in Bergmann Schaeffer Lehrbuch der Experimentalphysik. de Gruyter, Berlin, 7th edition, 1987.

[GW04a]   B. Gleich and J. Weizenecker. World Patent No. WO-2004091398-A2, April 2004.

[GW04b]   B. Gleich and J. Weizenecker. World Patent No. WO-2004091721-A1, April 2004.

[GW05]   B. Gleich and J. Weizenecker. Tomographic imaging using the nonlinear response of magnetic particles. *nature*, 435:1214–1217, 2005.

[GWB08]   B. Gleich, J. Weizenecker, and J. Borgert. Experimental results on fast 2D-encoded magnetic particle imaging. *Physics in Medicine and Biology*, 53(6):N81–N84, 2008.

[GWB10]   B. Gleich, J. Weizenecker, and J. Borgert. Acoustically detected Magnetic Particle Imaging, April 2010.

[GZL+06]   K. Golman, R. Zandt, M. Lerche, R. Pehrson, and J. Ardenkjaer-Larsen. Metabolic imaging by hyperpolarized 13C magnetic resonance imaging for in vivo tumor diagnosis. *Cancer Res.*, 66(22):10855–10860, 2006.

[HC05]   E. Hoffman and D. Chon. Computed tomography studies of lung ventilation and perfusion. *Proc Am Thorac Soc.*, 2(6):492–498, 2005.

[HHK98]   K. Hawkins, J. Henry, and R. Krasuski. Tissue harmonic imaging in echocardiography: better valve imaging, but at what cost? *Echocardiography*, 25(2):127–148, 1998.

[HHX08]   S. Haider, A. Hrbek, and Y. Xu. Magneto-acousto-electrical tomography: a potential method for imaging current densities and electrical impedance. *Physiol Meas.*, 29(6):S41–50, 2008.

[HKN87]   G. Harding, J. Kosanetzky, and U. Neitzel. X-ray diffraction computed tomography. *Med Phys*, 14(4):515–525, 1987.

[HMM+08]   F. Hyodo, R. Murugesan, K. Matsumoto, E. Hyodo, S. Subramanian, J. Mitchell, and M. Krishna. Monitoring redox-sensitive paramagnetic contrast agent by EPRI, OMRI and MRI. *J Magn Reson.*,, 190(1):105–112, 2008.

[Hou73]   G. Hounsfield. Computerized transverse axial scanning (tomography). 1. Description of system. *Br J Radiol.*, 46(552):1016–1022, 1973.

[How06]   D. Howarth. The role of nuclear medicine in the detection of acute gastrointestinal bleeding. *Semin Nucl Med.*, 36(2):133–146, 2006.

[HPKD03]   D. Hautot, Q. Pankhurst, N. Khan, and J. Dobson. Preliminary evaluation of nanoscale biogenic magnetite in Alzheimer's disease brain tissue. *Proc Biol Sci.*, 270(Suppl 1):S62–S64, 2003.

[HXT⁺02]   Y. He, D. Xing, S. Tan, Y. Tang, and K. Ueda. In vivo sonoluminiscence imaging with the assistance of FLAC. *Phys. Med. Biol.*, 47(9):1535–1541, 2002.

[JSH89]   M. Joy, G. Scott, and R. Henkelman. In-Vivo Detection of Applied Electric Currents by Magnetic Resonance Imaging, Magnetic Resonance Imaging. *Magnetic Resonance Imaging*, 7:89–94, 1989.

[JSR⁺93]   K. Joseph, J. Stapp, J. Reinecke, H. Skamel, H. Höffken, C. Neuhaus, H. Lenze, M. Trautmann, and R. Arnold. Receptor scintigraphy with 111In-pentetreotide for endocrine gastroenteropancreatic tumors. *Horm Metab Res Suppl.*, 27:28–35, 1993.

[JSW⁺97]   A. Jordan, R. Scholz, P. Wust, H. Fähling, J. Krause, W. Wlodarczyk, B. Sander, T. Vogl, and R. Felix. Effects of magnetic fluid hyperthermia (MFH) on C3H mammary carcinoma in vivo. *Int J Hyperthermia*, 13(6):587–605, 1997.

[KE63]   D. Kuhl and R. Edwards. Image separation radioisotope scanning. *Radiology*, 80:653, 1963.

[Kit86]   C. Kittel, editor. *Introduction to Solid State Physics.* John Wiley, New York, sixth edition, 1986.

[KMR⁺00]   R.A. Krueger, K.D. Miller, H.E. Reynolds, W.L. Kiser, D.R. Reinecke, and G.A. Krueger. Breast cancer in vivo: contrast enhancement with thermoacoustic CT at 434 MHz-feasibility study. *Radiology*, 216(1):279–283, 2000.

[Kne90]   F.K. Kneubühl. *Repetitorium der Physik,.* Teubner, Stuttgart, 1990. ISBN 3-519-33012-1.

[KYK97]   A. Kobayashi, N. Yamamoto, and J. Kirschvink. Studies of Inorganic Crystals in Biological Tissue: Magnetite in

Human Tumor. *Journal of the Japan Society of Powder Metallurgy*, 44:294–300, 1997.

[Lau73]   P. Lauterbur. Image Formation by Induced Local Interactions: Examples Employing Nuclear Magnetic Resonance. *nature*, 242:190–191, 1973.

[LBF⁺97]   R. Lawaczeck, H. Bauer, T. Frenzel, M. Hasegawa, Y. Ito, K. Kito, N. Miwa, H. Tsutsui, H. Vogler, and H. Weinmann. Magnetic iron oxide particles coated with carboxydextran for parenteral administration and liver contrasting. Pre-clinical profile of SH U555A. *Acta Radiol.*, 38(4 Pt 1):584–597, 1997.

[LBM98]   Y. Leroy, B. Bocquet, and A. Mamouni. Non-invasive microwave radiometry thermometry. *Physiol Meas.*, 19(2):127–148, 1998.

[LL99]   Z.-P. Liang and P. Lauterbur. *Principles of Magnetic Resonance Imaging: A Signal Processing Perspective*. Wiley-IEEE Press, 1999.

[LMB⁺99]   E. Lange, J. Mugler, J. Brookeman, J. Knight-Scott, J. Truwit, C. Teates, T. Daniel, P. Bogorad, and GD Cates. Lung air spaces: MR imaging evaluation with hyperpolarized 3He gas. *Radiology*, 210(3):861–857, 1999.

[MB07]   R. Moustafa and J. Baron. Clinical review: Imaging in ischaemic stroke–implications for acute management. *Crit Care.*, 11(5):227ff, 2007.

[MC93]   A. Macovski and S. Conolly. Novel approaches to low-cost MRI. *Magn Reson Med.*, 30(2):221–230, 1993.

[MH02]   J. Mayo and M. Hayden. Hyperpolarized helium 3 diffusion imaging of the lung. *Radiology*, 222(1):8–11, 2002.

[MHOS04]   R. Merwa, K. Hollaus, B. Oszkar, and H. Scharfetter. Detection of brain oedema using magnetic induction tomography: a feasibility study of the likely sensitivity and delectability. *Physiol. Meas.*, 25(1):347–354, 2004.

[Mor95]   H. Morneburg (Hrsg.), editor. *Bildgebende Systeme für die medizinische Diagnostik*. MDC Verlag, third edition, 1995.

[MRCBC08]   K. Mosbah, J. Ruiz-Cabello, Y. Berthezene, and Y. Cremillieux. Aerosols and gaseous contrast agents for magnetic resonance imaging of the lung. *Contrast Media Mol Imaging.*, 3(5):173–190, 2008.

[MTO+08]   J. Miyamoto, K. Tatsuzawa, K. Owada, T. Kawabe, H. Sasajima, and K. Mineura. Usefulness and limitations of fluorine-18-fluorodeoxyglucose positron emission tomography for the detection of malignancy of orbital tumors. *Neurol Med Chir (Tokyo)*, 48(11):495–499, 2008.

[MZX+05]   Y. Meng, M. Zhang, J. Xu, X. Liu, and Q. Ma. Effect of resveratrol on microcirculation disorder and lung injury following severe acute pancreatitis in rats. *World J Gastroenterol*, 11(3):433–435, 2005.

[NOB+86]   P. Nickers, L. Oosters, F. Brasseur, L. Deckers-Passau, and C. Deckers. Effect of chemotherapy on tumor temperature in rats. *Eur J Cancer Clin Oncol*, 22(4):381–385, 1986.

[OCF+80]   T. Ovitt, P. Christenson, H. Fisher, M. Frost, S. Nudelman, H. Roehrig, and G. Seeley. Intravenous angiography using digital video subtraction: x-ray imaging system. *AJR Am J Roentgeno*, 135(6):1141–1144, 1980.

[PAB00]   V. Passechnik, A. Anosov, and K. Bograchev. Fundamentals and Prospects of Passive Thermoacoustic Tomography. *Critical Reviews in Biomedical Engineering*, 28(3-4):349–357, 2000.

[PBH08]   K. Parodi, T. Bortfeld, and T. Haberer. Comparison between in-beam and offline positron emission tomography imaging of proton and carbon ion therapeutic irradiation at synchrotron- and cyclotron-based facilities. *Int. J. Radiat. Oncol. Biol. Phys.*, 71(3):945–956, 2008.

[PBSA92] K. Petrov, N. Borisenko, A. Starostin, and M. Alfimov. Polar Molecular Clustes Produced upon Photoinduced Electron Transfer in an Intermolecular Exciplex in Binary Solvents. *J. Phys. Chem*, 96:2091–2093, 1992.

[PHS+06] M. Peuster, C. Hesse, T. Schloo, C. Fink, P. Beerbaum, and C. Schnakenburg. Long-term biocompatibility of a corrodible peripheral iron stent in the porcine descending aorta. *Biomaterials*, 27(28):4955–4962, 2006.

[PMH+08] S. Patz, I. Muradian, M. Hrovat, I. Ruset, G. Topulos, S. Covrig, E. Frederick, H. Hatabu, F. Hersman, and J. Butler. Human pulmonary imaging and spectroscopy with hyperpolarized 129Xe at 0.2T. *Acad Radiol.*, 15(6):713–727, 2008.

[PSCLM07] J. Petersson, A. Sanchez-Crespo, S. Larsson, and M. Mure. Physiological imaging of the lung: single-photon-emission computed tomography (SPECT). *J Appl Physiol*, 102:468–476, 2007.

[PWSB99] K. Pruessmann, M. Weiger, M. Scheidegger, and P. Boesiger. SENSE: sensitivity encoding for fast MRI. *Magn Reson Med.*, 42(5):952–962, 1999.

[RBS+08] E. Roessl, B. Brendel, J. Schlomka, A Thran, and R. Proksa. Sensitivity of photon-counting k-edge imaging: Dependence on atomic number and object size. In *Nuclear Science Symposium Conference Record*, pages 4016–4021. IEEE, 2008.

[RBW94] B. Roth, P. Basser, and J. Wikswo. A theoretical model for magneto-acoustic imaging of bioelectric currents. *IEEE Trans Biomed Eng.*, 41(8):723–728, 1994.

[Rön96] C. Röntgen. Über eine neue art von strahlen, 1896.

[Rös87] P. Röschmann. Radiofrequency penetration and absorption in the human body: Limitations to high-field whole-body nuclear magnetic resonance imaging. *Med. Phys*, 14(6):922–931, 1987.

[SCM⁺01]   C. Stefanadis, C. Chrysochoou, D. Markou, K. Petraki, D. Panagiotakos, C. Fasoulakis, A. Kyriakidis, C. Papadimitriou, and P. Toutouzas. Increased temperature of malignant urinary bladder tumors in vivo: the application of a new method based on a catheter technique. *J Clin Oncol*, 19(3):676–681, 2001.

[SCP⁺03]   C. Stefanadis, C. Chrysohoou, D. Panagiotakos, E. Passalidou, V. Katsi, V. Polychronopoulos, and P. Toutouzas. Temperature differences are associated with malignancy on lung lesions: a clinical study. *BMC Cancer*, 3(1), 2003.

[SFK07]   K. Sakamoto, N. Furuya, and H Kanai. Optical characteristics of flowing blood: effects on the pulse oximeter. In *Conf Proc IEEE Eng Med Biol Soc*, pages 4552–4555. IEEE, 2007.

[SGB⁺06]   P. Smirnov, F. Gazeau, J. Beloeil, B. Doan, C. Wilhelm, and B. Gillet. Single-cell detection by gradient echo 9.4 T MRI: a parametric study. *Contrast Media Mol Imaging*, 1(4):165–174, 2006.

[SJAH95]   G. Scott, M. Joy, R. Armstrong, and R. Henkelman. Electromagnetic Considerations for RF Current Density Imaging. *IEEE Trans. Med. Imag.*, 14(3):515–524, 1995.

[SKB⁺09]   T. Sattel, T. Knopp, S. Biederer, B. Gleich, J. Weizenecker, J. Borgert, and T. Buzug. Single-Sided Device for Magnetic Particle Imaging. *Journal of Physics D: Applied Physics*, 42(2):1–5, 2009.

[SY08]   A. Sukstanskii and D. Yablonsky. In vivo lung morphometry with hyperpolarized 3He diffusion MRI: theoretical background. *J. Magn. Reson.*, 190(2):200–210, 2008.

[TOK08]   O.V. Trokhanova, M.B. Okhapkin, and A.V. Korjenevsky. Dual-frequency electrical impedance mammography for the diagnosis of non-malignant breast disease. *Physiol. Meas.*, 29(6):331–344, 2008.

[TPPHM75] M. Ter-Pogossian, M. Phelps, E. Hoffman, and N. Mullani. A positron-emission transaxial tomograph for nuclear imaging (PETT). *Radiology*, 114(1):89–98, 1975.

[UMH+06] S. Ungersma, N. Matter, J. Hardy, R. Venook, A. Macovski, S. Conolly, and G. Scott. Magnetic resonance imaging with T1 dispersion contrast. *Magn Reson Med.*, 55(6):1362–1371, 2006.

[VMR+06] R. Venook, N. Matter, M. Ramachandran, S. Ungersma, G. Gold, N. Giori, A. Macovski, G. Scott, and S. Conolly. Prepolarized magnetic resonance imaging around metal orthopedic implants. *Magn Reson Med.*, 56(1):177–86, 2006.

[WBG07] J. Weizenecker, J. Borgert, and B. Gleich. A simulation study on the resolution and sensitivity of magnetic particle imaging. *Physics in Medicine and Biology*, 52(21):6363–6374, 2007.

[WCC+07] P. Winter, K. Cai, S. Caruthers, S. Wickline, and G. Lanza. Emerging nanomedicine opportunities with perfluorocarbon nanoparticles. *Expert Rev Med Devices*, 4(2):137–145, 2007.

[WCK+99] W. Weitschies, D. Cardini, M. Karaus, L. Trahms, and W. Semmler. Magnetic marker monitoring of esophageal, gastric and duodenal transit of non-disintegrating capsules. *Pharmazie*, 54(6):426–430, 1999.

[WCY+06] J. Woods, C. Choong, D. Yablonsky, J. Bentley, J. Wong, J. Pierce, J. Cooper, P. Macklem, M. Conradi, and J. Hogg. Hyperpolarized 3HE diffusion MRI and histology in pulmonary emphysema. *Magn. Reson. Med.*, 56(6):1293–1300, 2006.

[WGB08] J. Weizenecker, B. Gleich, and J. Borgert. Magnetic particle imaging using a field free line. *J. Phys. D: Appl. Phys.*, 41:105009 (3pp), 2008.

[WGJ+06] P. Wust, U. Gneveckow, M. Johannsen, D. Böhmer, T. Henkel, F. Kahmann, J. Sehouli, R. Felix, J. Ricke, and A. Jordan. Magnetic nanoparticles for interstitial thermotherapy–feasibility, tolerance and achieved temperatures. *Int J Hyperthermia.*, 22(8):673–685, 2006.

[WGR⁺09] J. Weizenecker, B. Gleich, J. Rahmer, H. Dahnke, and J. Borgert. Three-dimensional real-time in-vivo magnetic particle imaging. *Physics in Medicine and Biology*, 54:L1–L10, 2009.

[WHS⁺77] S. Winkler, J. Holden, J. Sackett, D. Flemming, and S. Alexander. Xenon and krypton as radiographic inhalation contrast media with computerized tomography: preliminary note. *Invest Radiol*, 12(1):19–20, 1977.

[WKCT97] W. Weitschies, R. Kötitz, D. Cordini, and L. Trah. High resolution monitoring of the gastrointestinal transit of a magnetically marked capsule. *J Pharm*, 86:1218–1222, 1997.

[WMB⁺95] M. Weldon, A. Masoomi, A. Britten, J. Gane, C. Finlayson, A. Joseph, and J. Maxwell. Quantification of inflammatory bowel disease activity using technetium-99m HMPAO labelled leucocyte single photon emission computerised tomography (SPECT). *Gut*, 36(2):243–250, 1995.

[WS08] E. Woo and J. Seo. Magnetic resonance electrical impedance tomography (MREIT) for high-resolution conductivity imaging. *Physiol Meas.*, 29(10):R1–26, 2008.

[WTVF92] Press W., S. Teukolsky, W. Vetterling, and B. Flannery. *Numerical recipes in C : the art of scientific computing.* Cambridge University Press, Cambridge, second edition, 1992. ISBN 0521437202.

[YB05] X. Yuan and H. Bin. Magnetoacoustic Tomography with Magnetic Induction (MAT-MI). *Phys Med Biol.*, 50(21):5175–5187, 2005.

[YW00] G. Yao and L. Wang. heoretical and experimental studies of ultrasound-modulated optical tomography in biological tissue. *Appl. Opt.*, 39(4):59–664, 2000.

[ZLC⁺08]   Q. Zhang, Z. Liu, P.R. Carney, Z. Yuan, H. Chen, S. Roper, and H. Jiang. Non-invasive imaging of epileptic zeizures in vivo using photoacoustic tomogrophy. *Phys. Med. Biol.*, 53(7):1921–1931, 2008.

[ZOS⁺08]   S. Zink, S. Ohki, B. Stein, D. Zambuto, R. Rosenberg, J. Choi, and D. Tubbs. Noninvasive evaluation of active lower gastrointestinal bleeding: comparison between contrast-enhanced MDCT and 99mTc-labeled RBC scintigraphy. *AJR Am J Roentgenol*, 191(4), 2008.

[ZYS⁺05]   J. Zheng, Z. Yao, C. Shu, Y. Zhang, and X. Zhang. Role of SPECT/CT in diagnosis of hepatic hemangiomas. *World J Gastroenterol*, 11(34):5336–5341, 2005.

Aktuelle Forschung Medizintechnik

Herausgeber:

Prof. Dr. Thorsten M. Buzug

Institut für Medizintechnik, Universität zu Lübeck

Themen
Werke aus folgenden Themengebieten werden gerne in die Reihe aufgenommen: Biomedizinische Mikro- und Nanosysteme, Elektromedizin, biomedizinische Mess- und Sensortechnik, Monitoring, Lasertechnik, Robotik, minimalinvasive Chirurgie, integrierte OP-Systeme, bildgebende Verfahren, digitale Bildverarbeitung und Visualisierung, Kommunikations- und Informationssysteme, Telemedizin, eHealth und wissensbasierte Systeme, Biosignalverarbeitung, Modellierung und Simulation, Biomechanik, aktive und passive Implantate, Tissue Engineering, Neuroprothetik, Dosimetrie, Strahlenschutz, Strahlentherapie.

Autorinnen und Autoren
Autoren der Reihe sind in der Regel junge Promovierte und Habilitierte, die exzellente Abschlussarbeiten verfasst haben.

Leserschaft
Die Reihe wendet sich einerseits an Studierende, Promovenden und Habilitanden aus den Bereichen Medizintechnik, Medizinische Ingenieurwissenschaft, Medizinische Physik, Medizinische Informatik oder ähnlicher Richtungen. Andererseits stellt die Reihe aktuelle Arbeiten aus einem sich schnell entwickelnden Feld dar, so dass auch Wissenschaftlerinnen und Wissenschaftler sowie Entwicklerinnen und Entwickler an Universitäten, in außeruniversitären Forschungseinrichtungen und der Industrie von den ausgewählten Arbeiten in innovativen Gebieten der Medizintechnik profitieren werden.

Begutachtungsprozess
Die Qualitätssicherung erfolgt in drei Schritten. Zunächst werden nur Arbeiten angenommen die mindestens magna cum laude bewertet sind. Im zweiten Schritt wird ein Mitglied des Editorial Boards die Annahme oder Ablehnung des Werkes empfehlen. Im letzten Schritt wird der Reihenherausgeber über die Annahme oder Ablehnung entscheiden sowie Änderungen in der Druckfassung empfehlen. Die Koordination übernimmt der Reihenherausgeber.

Kontakt
Prof. Dr. Thorsten M. Buzug
Institut für Medizintechnik   Tel.:   +49 (0) 451 / 500-5400
Universität zu Lübeck   Fax: +49 (0) 451 / 500-5403
Ratzeburger Allee 160   E-Mail: buzug@imt.uni-luebeck.de
23538 Lübeck, Germany   Web: http://www.imt.uni-luebeck.de

Stand: Mai 2012. Änderungen vorbehalten.
Erhältlich im Buchhandel oder beim Verlag.

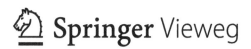 Springer Vieweg

Abraham-Lincoln-Straße 46
D-65189 Wiesbaden
Tel. +49 (0)6221. 345 - 4301
www.springer-vieweg.de